HANA KIM

Low-FODMAP Cookbook for a Healthier You

Managing Irritable Bowel Syndrome with Simple and Delicious Recipes

Contents

Conclusion

Acknowledgement

Creating the "Low-FODMAP Cookbook for a Healthier You" has been a journey filled with learning, creativity, and collaboration. I am deeply grateful to everyone who has contributed to making this book a reality.

First and foremost, I want to express my heartfelt thanks to the researchers at Monash University. Their pioneering work on the low-FODMAP diet has transformed the lives of countless people with IBS, including myself. Your dedication to improving the understanding and management of this condition is truly inspiring.

To the medical professionals and dietitians who provided their expertise and support, thank you for your invaluable contributions. Your insights ensured that this cookbook is not only delicious but also scientifically sound and beneficial for those managing IBS.

A special thank you to my recipe testers and taste-testers. Your feedback, patience, and enthusiasm were essential in perfecting these recipes. I am especially grateful to those who live with IBS and took the time to test these recipes in their own kitchens. Your input helped shape a cookbook that is both practical and effective.

To my editor and publishing team, your guidance and hard work have been instrumental in bringing this book to life. Thank you for your meticulous attention to detail and for believing in this project.

To my friends and family, your unwavering support and encouragement have been my anchor throughout this journey. Thank you for understanding the late nights and for being my constant source of motivation.

Lastly, to the readers, thank you for trusting me to guide you on your low-FODMAP journey. Your health and well-being are at the heart of this book, and I hope it brings you relief and joy in the kitchen. Your stories and experiences inspire me every day, and I am honored to be a part of your journey towards a healthier, happier life.

With gratitude,

Hana Kim.

Introduction

Welcome to the "Low-FODMAP Cookbook for a Healthier You: Managing Irritable Bowel Syndrome with Simple and Delicious Recipes." If you've picked up this book, chances are you or someone you love is dealing with the daily challenges of Irritable Bowel Syndrome (IBS). You're not alone—IBS affects millions of people worldwide, causing symptoms that can significantly impact your quality of life. But there is hope, and this cookbook is here to provide a practical and tasty solution.

The low-FODMAP diet, developed by researchers at Monash University, has emerged as a highly effective approach to managing IBS symptoms. This diet involves reducing the intake of certain carbohydrates known as FODMAPs (Fermentable Oligo-, Di-, Mono-saccharides and Polyols), which are poorly absorbed in the small intestine and can cause discomfort in people with IBS. By following a low-FODMAP diet, many people have found significant relief from symptoms such as bloating, gas, stomach pain, and irregular bowel movements.

In this cookbook, you will find a wealth of information and resources to help you embark on your low-FODMAP journey. Whether you're newly diagnosed with IBS or have been struggling for years, this book is designed to be your companion in the kitchen and beyond. We have organized the content into three main parts to guide you through understanding IBS and the low-FODMAP diet, enjoying delicious low-FODMAP recipes, and integrating this lifestyle into your daily routine.

Part 1: Introduction to Low-FODMAP and IBS

This section provides a comprehensive overview of IBS and the low-FODMAP diet. You will learn about the science behind FODMAPs, how they affect your digestive system, and why this diet can be beneficial. We'll guide you through the initial phases of the diet, including the elimination and reintroduction stages, to help you identify your personal triggers and develop a sustainable eating plan.

Part 2: Low-FODMAP Recipes

The heart of this cookbook lies in its recipes. We've curated a variety of simple, tasty, and nutritious dishes that are all low-FODMAP. From breakfast to dinner, including snacks and desserts, you'll find something for every meal and occasion. These recipes are designed not only to be gut-friendly but also to please your taste buds and make mealtime enjoyable again.

Part 3: Living with Low-FODMAP

Adopting a low-FODMAP lifestyle goes beyond just what you eat. In this section, we provide practical tips for dining out, traveling, and managing social situations while sticking to your diet. You'll also find strategies for maintaining long-term success, coping with setbacks, and supporting your overall gut health through stress management and other holistic approaches.

Our goal is to empower you with the knowledge and tools to take control of your IBS symptoms and improve your quality of life. We believe that eating low-FODMAP doesn't have to be restrictive or bland. With the right guidance and a bit of creativity, you can enjoy a diverse and flavorful diet that supports your health and well-being.

So, let's get started on this journey to a healthier, happier you. Turn the page, and let's cook up some delicious, low-FODMAP meals together!

With warmth and encouragement,

Hana Kim.

I

Introduction to Low-FODMAP and IBS

Understanding Irritable Bowel Syndrome (IBS)

A Frustrating But Common Foe

Have you ever dreamt of wearing that cute new outfit, only to have your stomach erupt in a symphony of gurgling and bloating? Or maybe that delicious work lunch leaves you glued to your chair, fearing the next bathroom dash? If so, you might be one of the millions of people worldwide living with a frustrating companion known as Irritable Bowel Syndrome, or IBS.

What is IBS?

IBS is a functional bowel disorder, meaning there's no visible damage to the gut, but its function is disrupted. It can feel like a constant shadow, an uninvited guest at every meal and a party pooper for any social plans.

While the exact cause of IBS remains a mystery, it's thought to be a combination of factors, including:

- **Gut sensitivity:** People with IBS may have a more sensitive gut that reacts more intensely to certain foods, stress, or hormonal changes.
- **Abnormal gut motility:** The muscles in the gut may contract too frequently or not forcefully enough, leading to constipation or diarrhea.
- **Microbiome imbalance:** The delicate balance of bacteria in the gut may be disrupted, contributing to digestive issues.

The IBS Rollercoaster: Common Symptoms and Their Impact

IBS symptoms can vary from person to person, but some common culprits include:

- **Bloating:** That uncomfortable feeling of a balloon inflating in your abdomen can be a constant source of discomfort and self-consciousness.
- **Cramping:** Sharp pains or dull aches that double you over can disrupt your daily activities and leave you constantly on edge.
- **Diarrhea or constipation:** Unpredictable bathroom urgency or difficulty passing stool can be a major inconvenience and source of anxiety, especially in social situations.
- **Gas:** Excessive gas and bloating can be not only uncomfortable but also embarrassing.
- **Fatigue:** IBS can leave you feeling drained and exhausted, impacting your energy levels and overall well-being.

These symptoms can wreak havoc on your daily life. Imagine the frustration of canceling plans because of a sudden IBS flare-up, or the constant worry about having access to a bathroom. IBS can affect your work, social life, and overall sense of control.

Traditional Treatments: Seeking Relief, But Not Always Finding It

There's currently no cure for IBS, but traditional treatments aim to manage symptoms. These may include:

- **Dietary changes:** Doctors may recommend a general low-fiber diet or eliminating specific triggers like caffeine or dairy. While this can be helpful for some, it often involves a lot of trial and error without a guaranteed solution.
- **Medication:** Antispasmodics can help relieve cramping, while antidiarrheals or laxatives can address constipation or diarrhea. However, these medications can come with side effects and may not address the root cause of the problem.
- **Therapy:** Stress management techniques like cognitive behavioral therapy can be helpful, as stress is often a trigger for IBS symptoms. But this

doesn't address the underlying gut issues.

While traditional treatments can offer some relief, many people with IBS find them to be limited or ineffective. They may still experience frequent flare-ups and feel restricted in their dietary choices. This can be incredibly frustrating and leave you searching for a better solution.

A New Hope: The Low-FODMAP Diet as an Alternative Approach

There's a ray of light at the end of the IBS tunnel! A revolutionary approach called the low-FODMAP diet is emerging as a game-changer for many IBS sufferers. This diet focuses on identifying and temporarily restricting specific types of carbohydrates that can be poorly absorbed in the gut, leading to those uncomfortable IBS symptoms. We'll delve deeper into the science behind low-FODMAP in the next chapter, but for now, know that it offers a more targeted approach to managing your gut health and potentially reducing IBS symptoms.

This chapter has just scratched the surface of IBS. The good news is, there's hope! In the following chapters, we'll explore the science behind the low-FODMAP diet, equip you with the tools to get started, and guide you on a delicious and empowering journey to a happier, healthier gut.

The Science Behind Low-FODMAP

Imagine your gut as a bustling city with tiny highways for food particles to travel. These highways are lined with hardworking transporters that unload deliveries of nutrients from your food. But what if there were certain types of cargo that some transporters struggled to handle? This is where FODMAPs come in, and where the science behind the low–FODMAP diet gets fascinating.

FODMAPs: The Culprits Behind the Chaos?

FODMAP is an acronym for a group of fermentable oligosaccharides, disaccharides, monosaccharides, and polyols. Let's break that down:

- **Oligosaccharides and disaccharides:** These are types of sugars that are chains of sugar molecules linked together. Fructans (found in wheat and rye) and lactose (milk sugar) are examples.
- **Monosaccharides:** These are single sugar molecules, like fructose (found in fruits) and excess free fructose (sometimes found in processed foods with high-fructose corn syrup).
- **Polyols:** These are sugar alcohols that are poorly absorbed by the gut, such as sorbitol (found in some fruits and artificial sweeteners).

For people with IBS, these FODMAPs can be problematic. They may not be fully absorbed by the small intestine, leading to a traffic jam in the gut. This can cause:

- **Fermentation:** Bacteria in the gut feed on these unabsorbed FODMAPs, producing gas as a byproduct. This gas can cause bloating, cramping, and discomfort.

- **Osmotic effects:** FODMAPs draw water into the gut, which can lead to diarrhea or loose stools.

The Low-FODMAP Diet: A Targeted Approach

The low-FODMAP diet is a three-phase approach designed to target these FODMAP culprits and potentially reduce IBS symptoms.

- **Phase 1: Elimination (6-8 weeks):** During this phase, you temporarily restrict high-FODMAP foods. Think of it as a highway closure for essential repairs. This allows your gut to heal and inflammation to subside.
- **Phase 2: Reintroduction (up to 8 weeks):** Here's where the detective work begins! We slowly reintroduce FODMAP groups one at a time, like carefully testing each lane of traffic. This helps you identify which specific FODMAPs might be causing problems in your own unique gut.
- **Phase 3: Maintaining a Low-FODMAP Lifestyle:** With your personalized knowledge of FODMAP triggers, you can create a sustainable, long-term eating plan that keeps your gut happy and symptoms under control.

Benefits Beyond Symptom Relief: A Healthier You

The low-FODMAP diet isn't just about reducing bloating and cramping. Studies have shown it to be highly effective in reducing a variety of IBS symptoms, including:

- **Pain and cramping**
- **Diarrhea and constipation**
- **Bloating and gas**
- **Overall gut discomfort**

But the benefits may extend beyond symptom relief. By promoting a healthier gut environment, the low-FODMAP diet may also contribute to:

- **Improved gut health:** A balanced gut microbiome with reduced inflammation can lead to better overall health and digestion.
- **Enhanced energy levels:** Reduced gut issues can improve nutrient absorption and leave you feeling more energized.
- **Increased quality of life:** When you're free from constant IBS flare-ups, you can enjoy life more fully and participate in activities without worry.

The science behind low-FODMAP is compelling. It offers a personalized approach to managing IBS and potentially unlocking a healthier, happier you. In the next chapter, we'll equip you with the tools and knowledge to get started on your low-FODMAP journey.

Getting Started with the Low-FODMAP Diet

So, you're ready to embark on the exciting journey of the low-FODMAP diet! This chapter will be your essential guide, equipping you with the tools and knowledge to navigate your low-FODMAP kitchen with confidence.

Building Your Low-FODMAP Pantry: Essential Staples

Imagine your pantry as your new low-FODMAP headquarters. Here, you'll stock up on gut-friendly ingredients that will form the foundation of your delicious and healthy meals. Let's take a tour of some key staples:

- **Low-FODMAP Fruits:** Berries, grapes, oranges, kiwi, and cantaloupe are some fantastic choices. These fruits provide essential vitamins, minerals, and natural sweetness.
- **Low-FODMAP Vegetables:** Get creative with a rainbow of low-FODMAP veggies like leafy greens, eggplant, zucchini, carrots, and bell peppers. They'll add vibrant colors, nutrients, and fiber to your meals.
- **Proteins:** Low-FODMAP protein sources like lean meats, poultry, fish, eggs, and tofu will keep you feeling satisfied and provide essential building blocks for your body.
- **Grains and Starches:** While some grains are high in FODMAPs, there are still plenty of options! Stock up on quinoa, rice, gluten-free oats, and low-FODMAP flours for baking.
- **Dairy Alternatives:** If you're sensitive to lactose, don't worry! Lactose-

free milk, yogurt, and cheese will provide essential calcium and creamy textures without the discomfort.

- **Healthy Fats:** Include heart-healthy fats like olive oil, avocado oil, nuts (in moderation), and seeds in your diet. They'll add flavor, richness, and essential nutrients.

Decoding Food Labels: Your Low-FODMAP Shopping Companion

Food labels can be like a foreign language, but fret not! Here are some tips for navigating them on your low-FODMAP journey:

- **Ingredients List:** This is your best friend! Scan the list for high-FODMAP ingredients like wheat, rye, milk, and certain fruits like apples and mangoes. Look for low-FODMAP alternatives or choose products labeled "lactose-free" or "gluten-free" when needed.
- **Serving Size:** Be mindful of portion sizes. Even low-FODMAP foods can become problematic if you eat too much at once. Pay attention to serving sizes and adjust as needed.
- **FODMAP Apps and Resources:** Consider using a reliable FODMAP app or online resource to help you identify low-FODMAP products and navigate tricky ingredients.

Stocking Up for Success: Tips for a Low-FODMAP Kitchen

- **Declutter and Clean Out:** Before embracing your new low-FODMAP staples, take some time to declutter your pantry and fridge. Remove any high-FODMAP foods that might tempt you during the elimination phase.
- **Invest in Low-FODMAP Staples:** Stock up on the essential low-FODMAP ingredients we discussed earlier. Having these readily available will make meal planning and cooking a breeze.
- **Plan Your Meals:** Spend some time planning your meals and snacks for the week. This will help you avoid last-minute decisions that might lead to unhealthy choices. There are plenty of low-FODMAP recipe resources available online and in cookbooks to inspire you.

Starting a New Journey: Encouragement and Support

We know starting a new diet can be daunting. But remember, you're not alone! Here are some words of encouragement to keep you motivated:

- **Focus on the Positive:** Instead of dwelling on what you can't eat, focus on the delicious and healthy low-FODMAP options that await you. Explore new recipes, experiment with flavors, and discover the joy of gut-friendly cooking.
- **Celebrate Small Wins:** Every step forward is a victory! Track your progress, celebrate milestones, and acknowledge the positive changes you're experiencing in your gut health and overall well-being.
- **Connect with the Low-FODMAP Community:** There are online forums, support groups, and social media communities dedicated to low-FODMAP living. Connect with others on the journey, share experiences, and gain valuable inspiration.

Remember, the low-FODMAP diet is a journey, not a destination. There will be challenges and moments of temptation, but with the right tools, knowledge, and support system, you can empower yourself to take control of your gut health and unlock a happier, healthier you.

II

Low-FODMAP Recipes

The rumble in your tummy isn't about to be silenced by bland, boring food! Part 2 of your low-FODMAP adventure is all about transforming your diet into a flavor fiesta. We'll be your guide, whipping up a delightful array of recipes that are both gut-friendly and incredibly satisfying.

Breakfast

Sunshine Smoothie Bowl

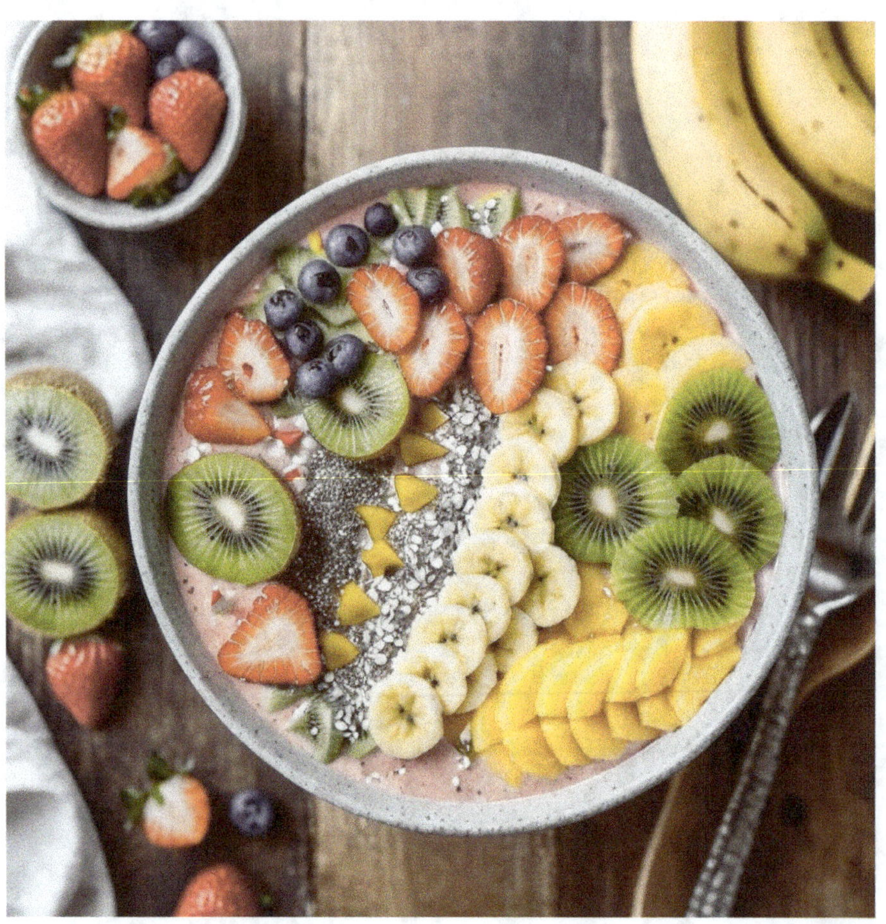

- **Yields:** 1 serving
- **Prep Time:** 5 minutes
- **Cook Time:** N/A
- **Total Time:** 5 minutes

Ingredients:

- 1/2 cup lactose-free yogurt
- 1/2 banana, frozen
- 1/2 cup chopped pineapple

- 1/4 cup packed baby spinach
- 1/4 cup unsweetened almond milk
- Drizzle of honey (optional)
- Toppings (optional): sliced strawberries, chia seeds, chopped nuts

Instructions:

1. Combine all ingredients in a blender. Blend until smooth and creamy, scraping down the sides as needed.
2. Pour into a bowl and top with your favorite low-FODMAP toppings.

Serving Suggestion:

Enjoy this vibrant smoothie bowl for a refreshing and energizing breakfast.

Notes:

- You can substitute the almond milk with another low-FODMAP milk alternative like lactose-free milk or rice milk.
- Feel free to adjust the sweetness to your preference by adding more or less honey.

* * *

Fluffy Scrambled Eggs with Spinach and Mushrooms

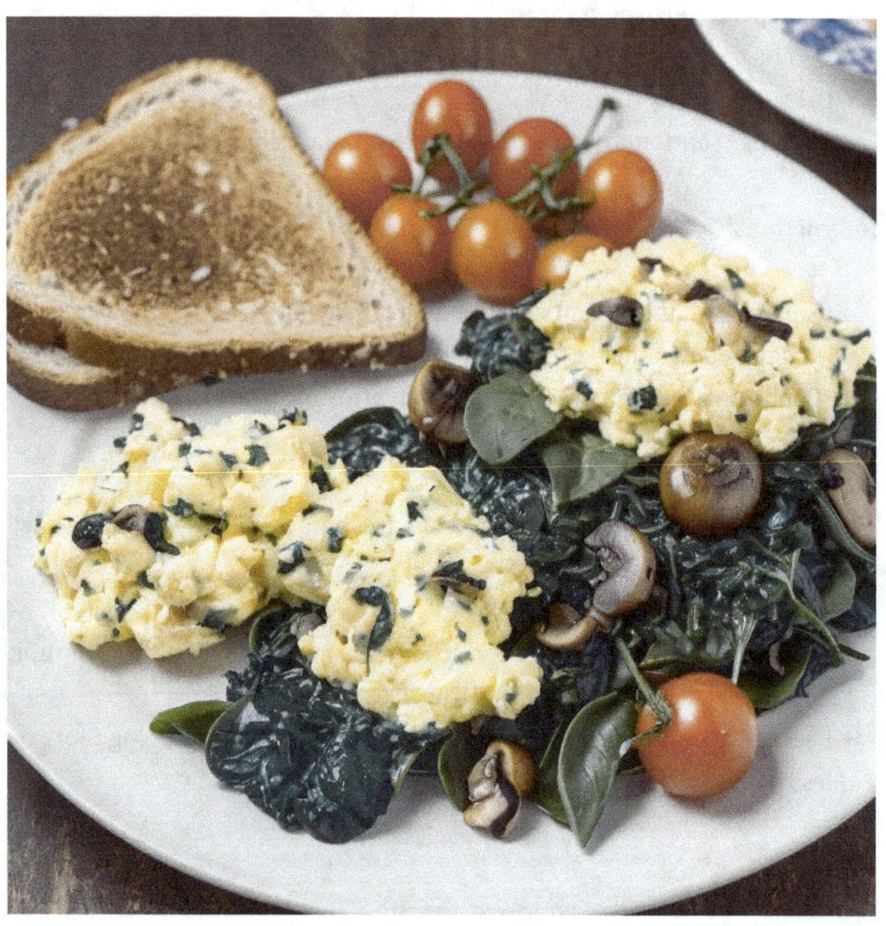

- **Yields:** 1 serving
- **Prep Time:** 5 minutes
- **Cook Time:** 5 minutes
- **Total Time:** 10 minutes

Ingredients:

- 2 eggs
- 1 tablespoon lactose-free milk

- 1 tablespoon olive oil
- ½ cup chopped spinach
- ½ cup sliced mushrooms
- Salt and pepper to taste

Instructions:

1. Whisk together eggs and lactose-free milk in a bowl. Season with salt and pepper.
2. Heat olive oil in a pan over medium heat. Add the mushrooms and cook until softened, about 3 minutes.
3. Add the spinach and cook until wilted, about 1 minute.
4. Pour in the egg mixture and gently stir with a spatula until the eggs are cooked through and fluffy, about 3-4 minutes.

Serving Suggestion:

Serve immediately with a slice of gluten-free toast for dipping.

Notes:

- For a richer flavor, you can add a sprinkle of grated Parmesan cheese (optional) just before the eggs are fully cooked.

* * *

Berry Bliss Chia Pudding

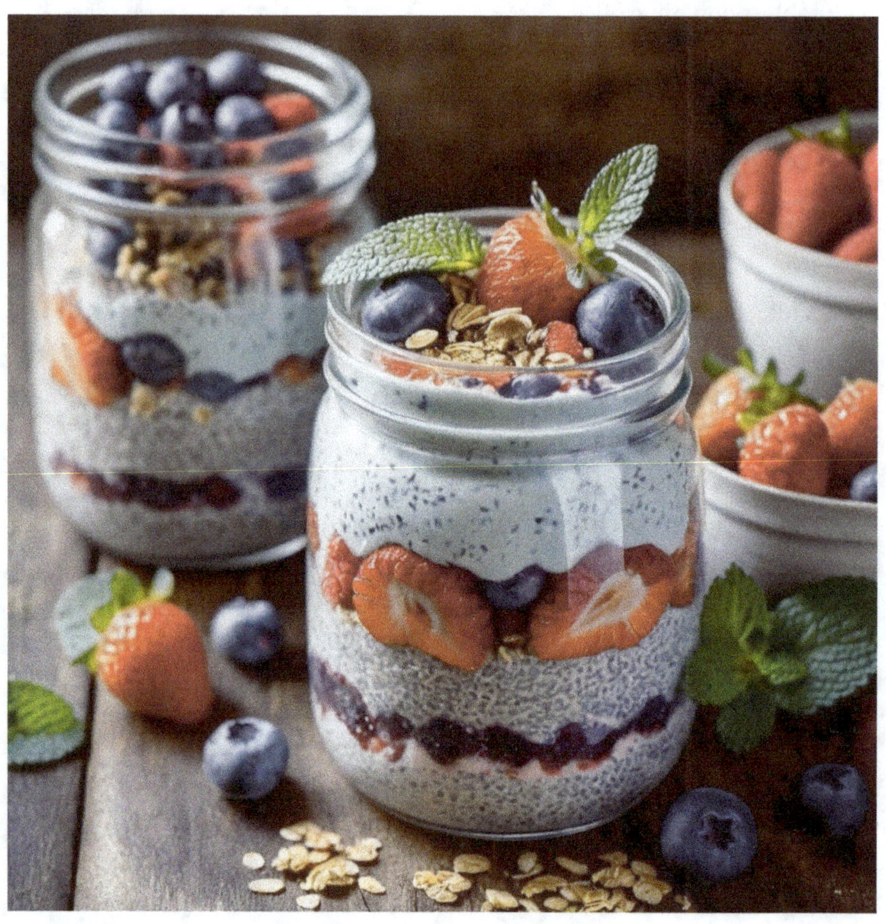

- **Yields:** 1 serving
- **Prep Time:** 5 minutes (plus overnight chilling)
- **Cook Time:** N/A
- **Total Time:** 5 minutes + overnight chilling

Ingredients:

- ¼ cup chia seeds
- ¾ cup lactose-free milk

- 1 tablespoon maple syrup
- ½ cup blueberries
- ½ cup raspberries

Instructions:

1. In a jar, combine chia seeds, lactose-free milk, and maple syrup. Stir well.
2. Fold in the blueberries and raspberries.
3. Cover the jar and refrigerate overnight, or at least for 4 hours, to allow the chia seeds to absorb the liquid and thicken.

Serving Suggestion:

Enjoy cold in the morning, or top with additional berries and a sprinkle of sliced almonds.

Notes:

- Feel free to adjust the amount of maple syrup to your preference.
- You can substitute other low-FODMAP fruits like chopped mango or sliced strawberries for the berries.

* * *

Savory Quinoa Breakfast Bowl

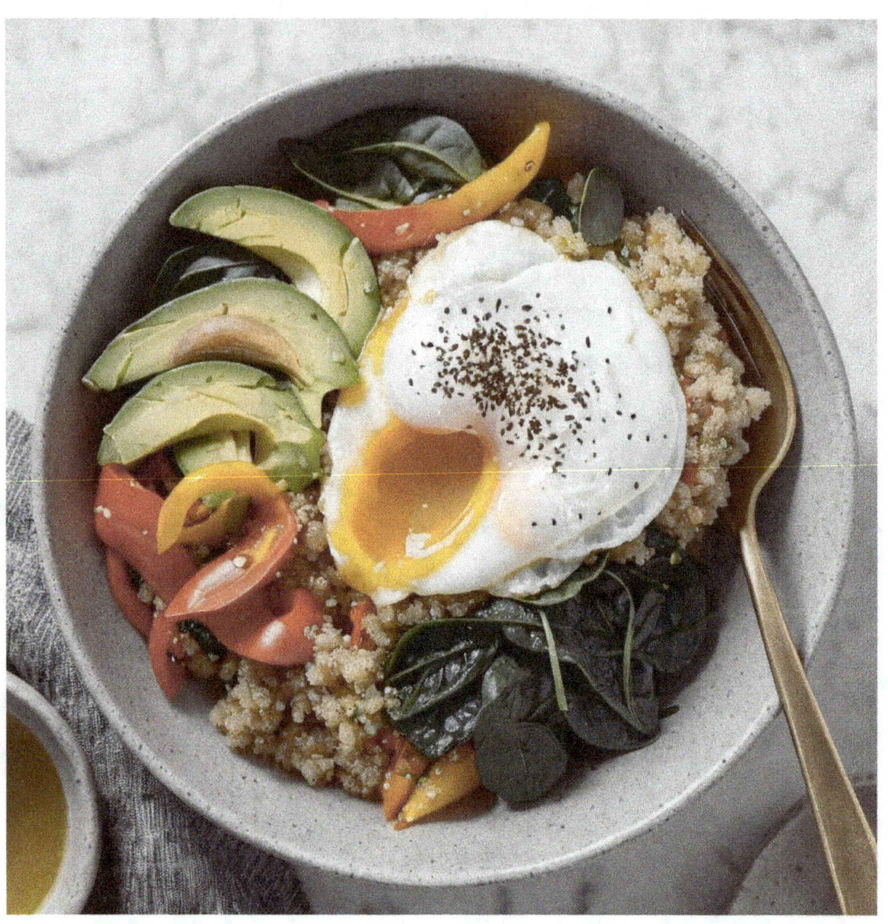

- **Yields:** 1 serving
- **Prep Time:** 5 minutes (plus cook time for quinoa)
- **Cook Time:** (refer to quinoa package instructions)
- **Total Time:** 5 minutes + quinoa cook time

Ingredients:

- 1 cup cooked quinoa
- 1 hard-boiled egg, sliced

- ½ avocado, diced
- ½ cup cherry tomatoes, diced
- 1 tablespoon olive oil
- 1 tablespoon lemon juice
- Salt and pepper to taste

Instructions:

1. Cook quinoa according to package directions.
2. In a bowl, combine cooked quinoa, sliced egg, diced avocado, and cherry tomatoes.
3. In a small bowl, whisk together olive oil and lemon juice. Drizzle over the quinoa mixture and toss to coat.
4. Season with salt and pepper to taste.

Serving Suggestion:

Serve immediately for a protein and fiber-rich breakfast bowl.

Notes:

- You can add a sprinkle of chopped fresh herbs like parsley or cilantro for extra flavor.
- Leftovers can be stored in an airtight container in the refrigerator for up to 2 days.

* * *

Tropical Frittata

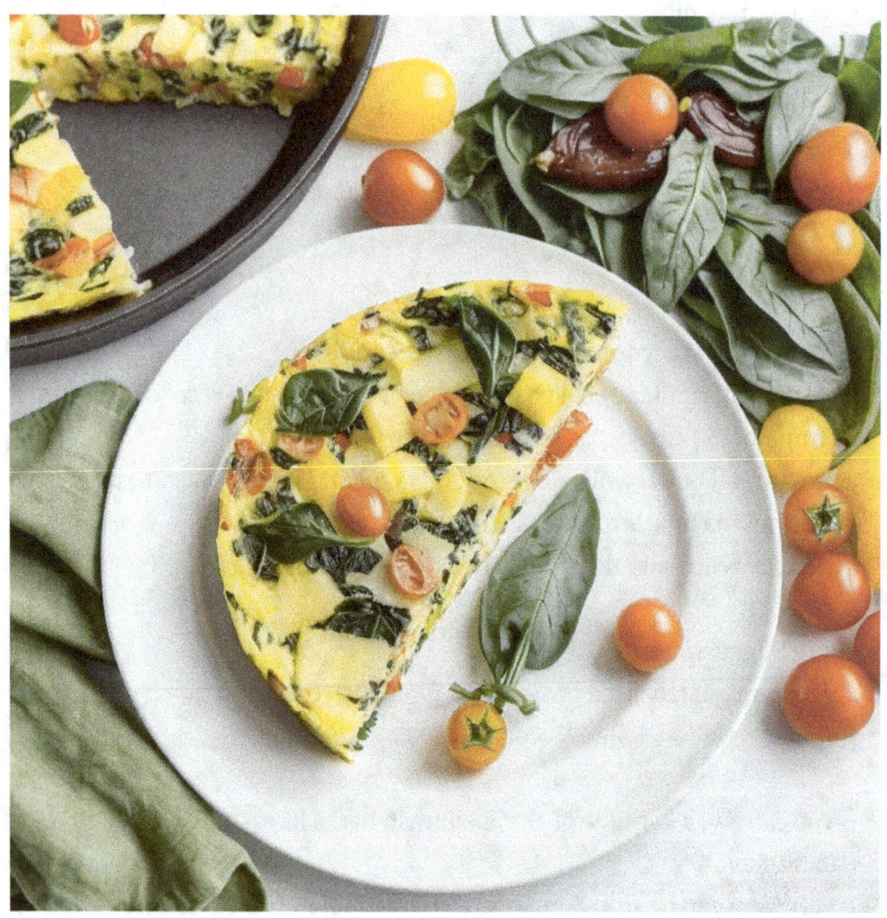

- **Yields:** 4 servings
- **Prep Time:** 10 minutes
- **Cook Time:** 20 minutes
- **Total Time:** 30 minutes

Ingredients:

- 1 tablespoon olive oil
- ½ cup chopped bell peppers (red, yellow, or orange)

- ½ cup sliced zucchini
- ½ cup cherry tomatoes
- 6 eggs
- ¼ cup lactose-free milk or milk alternative
- ¼ cup grated Parmesan cheese (optional)
- Salt and pepper to taste
- Fresh chopped parsley (optional, for garnish)

Instructions:

1. Preheat oven to 375°F (190°C). Grease a small oven-safe skillet or baking dish.
2. Heat olive oil in a pan over medium heat. Add bell peppers, zucchini, and cherry tomatoes. Sauté for 5-7 minutes, or until softened.
3. In a bowl, whisk together eggs, lactose-free milk, and Parmesan cheese (if using). Season with salt and pepper.
4. Pour the egg mixture over the vegetables in the prepared skillet.
5. Bake in the preheated oven for 20-25 minutes, or until the eggs are set and the center is no longer runny.
6. Garnish with fresh chopped parsley (optional) and serve warm.

Serving Suggestion:

Enjoy a slice of warm frittata for a satisfying breakfast. You can serve it with a side of gluten-free toast or a salad.

Notes:

- Feel free to add other low-FODMAP vegetables to the frittata, such as chopped mushrooms or spinach.
- Leftovers can be stored in an airtight container in the refrigerator for up to 3 days.

* * *

Simple Sweet Potato Pancakes

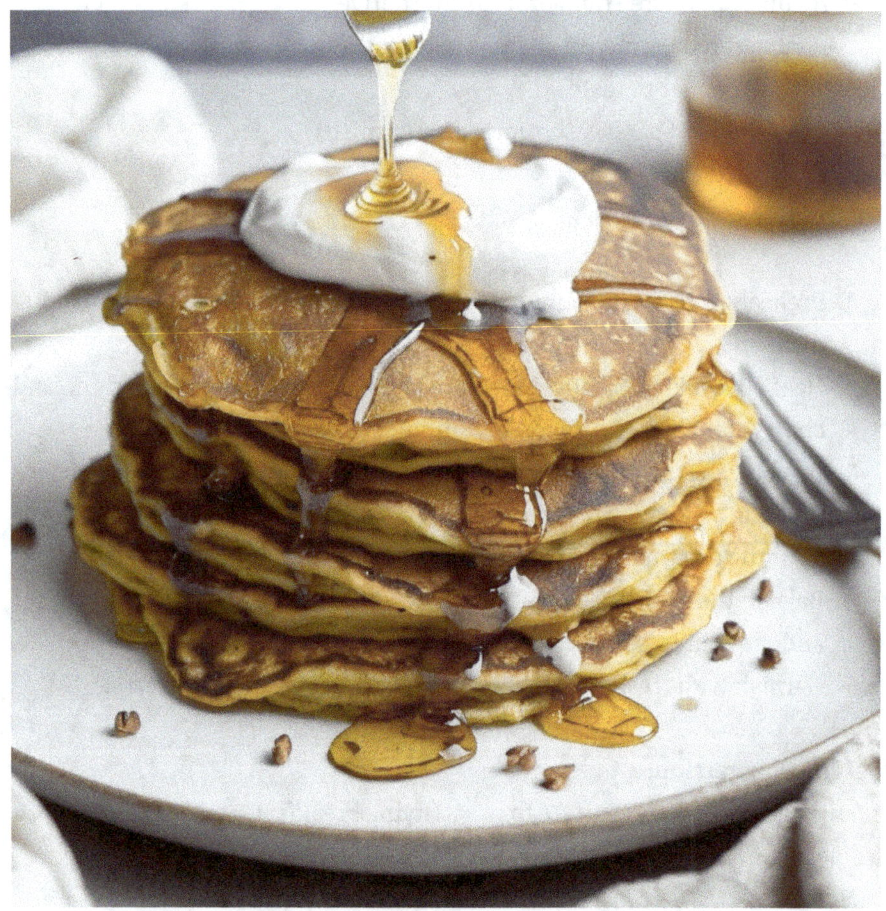

- **Yields:** 2-3 pancakes
- **Prep Time:** 10 minutes
- **Cook Time:** 5 minutes per side
- **Total Time:** 15 minutes

Ingredients:

- 1 medium sweet potato, grated
- 1 egg
- 1 tablespoon almond milk
- ½ teaspoon ground cinnamon
- ¼ teaspoon ground nutmeg
- Coconut oil or olive oil, for cooking

Instructions:

1. Grate the sweet potato using a box grater. Squeeze out any excess moisture with a paper towel or clean kitchen cloth.
2. In a bowl, combine grated sweet potato, egg, almond milk, cinnamon, and nutmeg. Mix well.
3. Heat a pan or griddle over medium heat. Add a drizzle of coconut oil or olive oil.
4. Pour ¼ cup batter per pancake onto the hot pan. Cook for 3-4 minutes per side, or until golden brown and cooked through.
5. Flip the pancakes carefully using a spatula and cook for an additional 2-3 minutes on the other side.

Serving Suggestion:
Serve warm with your favorite low-FODMAP toppings, such as sliced banana, chopped nuts, or a drizzle of maple syrup.

Notes:

- The amount of batter you get will depend on the size of your sweet potato. You may need to adjust the cooking time slightly depending on the thickness of your pancakes.
- Leftovers can be stored in an airtight container in the refrigerator for up to 2 days. Reheat gently in a pan or toaster oven.

* * *

Creamy Coconut Rice Porridge

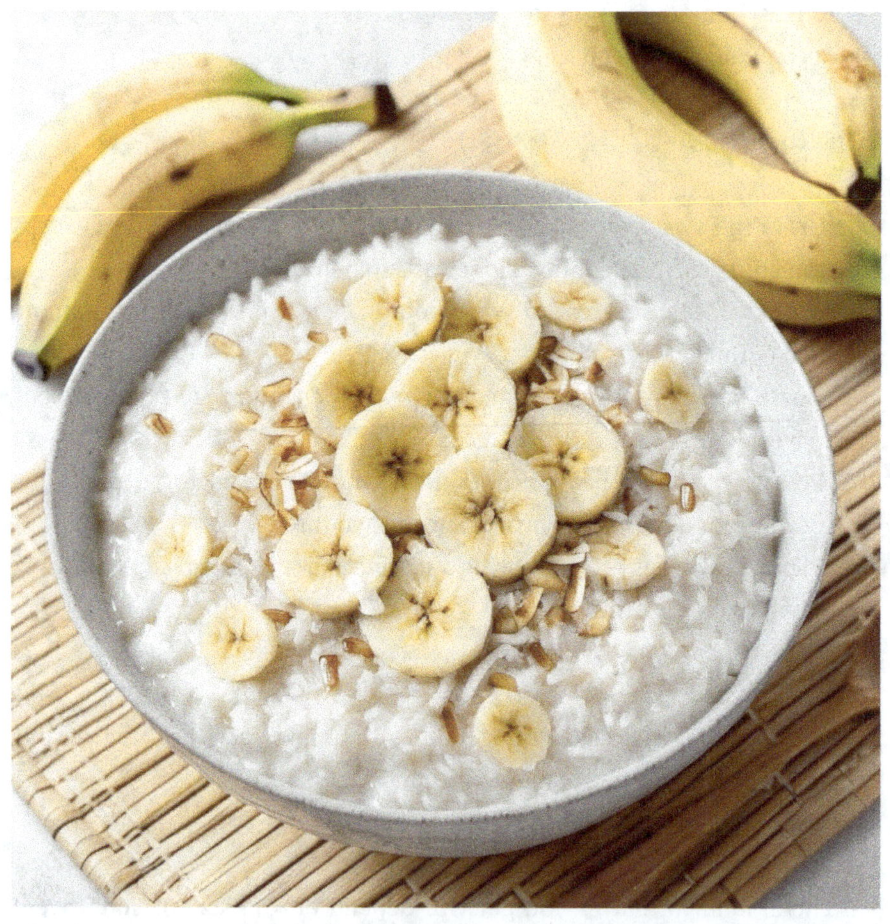

- **Yields:** 1 serving
- **Prep Time:** 5 minutes

- **Cook Time:** 15 minutes
- **Total Time:** 20 minutes

Ingredients:

- ½ cup chopped green banana (limited amount)
- ¾ cup canned coconut milk
- ½ teaspoon ground cinnamon
- ¼ teaspoon ground ginger
- 2 tablespoons rolled oats
- Toppings (optional): sliced strawberries, chopped coconut

Instructions:

1. In a saucepan, combine chopped green banana, coconut milk, cinnamon, and ginger.
2. Bring to a simmer over medium heat. Cook for 5 minutes, or until the green banana is softened.
3. Using a fork or potato masher, mash the green banana into the coconut milk to create a creamy consistency.
4. Stir in the rolled oats and cook for an additional 5-7 minutes, or until the oats are softened and the porridge thickens slightly.
5. Remove from heat and let cool slightly.

Serving Suggestion:

Pour the porridge into a bowl and top with sliced strawberries and chopped coconut (optional). Enjoy warm for a comforting and delicious breakfast.

Notes:

- Be sure to use green bananas for this recipe, as ripe bananas are high in FODMAPs.
- You can adjust the thickness of the porridge by adding more or less coconut milk.

- Leftovers can be stored in an airtight container in the refrigerator for up to 2 days.

* * *

Low-FODMAP Breakfast Burrito

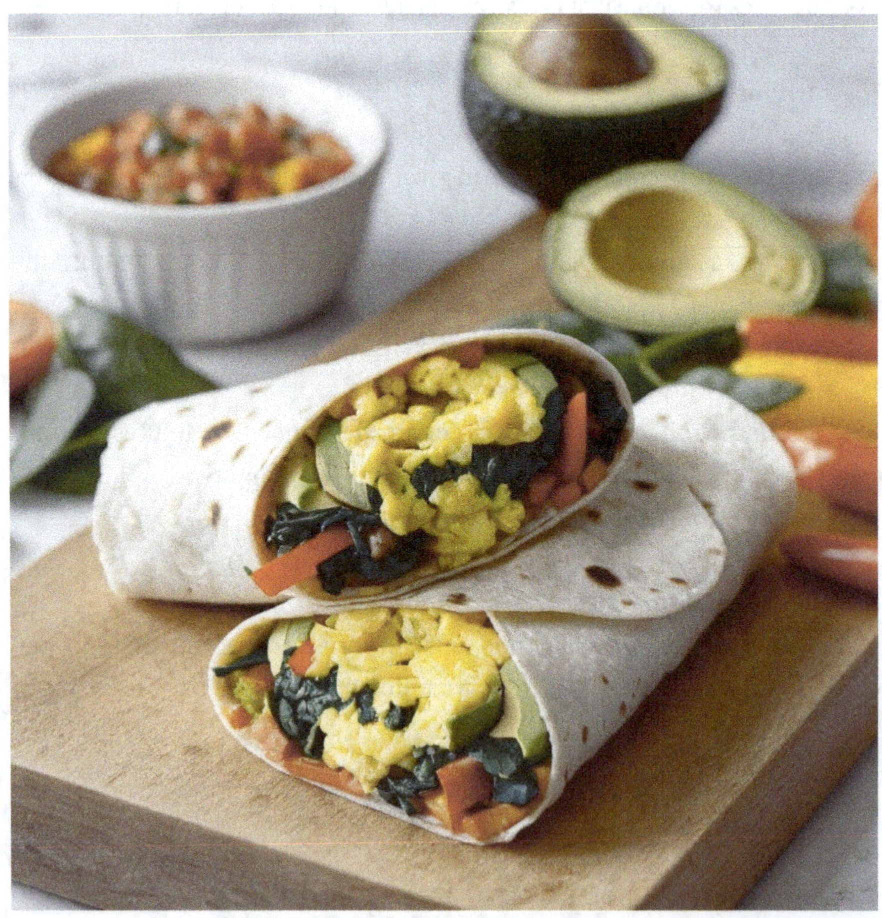

- **Yields:** 1 serving
- **Prep Time:** 5 minutes
- **Cook Time:** 5 minutes
- **Total Time:** 10 minutes

Ingredients:

- 2 eggs
- ½ cup chopped spinach
- ½ cup diced bell peppers (red, yellow, or orange)
- 1 gluten-free tortilla
- ¼ cup diced avocado
- Salsa (low-FODMAP option)
- Salt and pepper to taste

Instructions:

1. Scramble the eggs in a pan with a drizzle of olive oil. Season with salt and pepper.
2. While the eggs are cooking, stir in the chopped spinach and diced bell peppers. Cook until the spinach is wilted and the peppers are softened.
3. Warm a gluten-free tortilla in a dry pan or microwave for a few seconds.
4. Spread the scrambled egg mixture onto the warmed tortilla. Top with diced avocado and salsa.
5. Fold the tortilla into a burrito shape and enjoy!

Serving Suggestion:
Enjoy this protein and veggie-packed breakfast burrito for a quick and satisfying on-the-go meal.

Notes:

- Feel free to add other low-FODMAP vegetables to the burrito, such as chopped mushrooms or cherry tomatoes.

· You can also add a sprinkle of your favorite low–FODMAP cheese (optional) to the scrambled eggs for extra flavor.

* * *

Hearty Nut Butter and Banana Toast

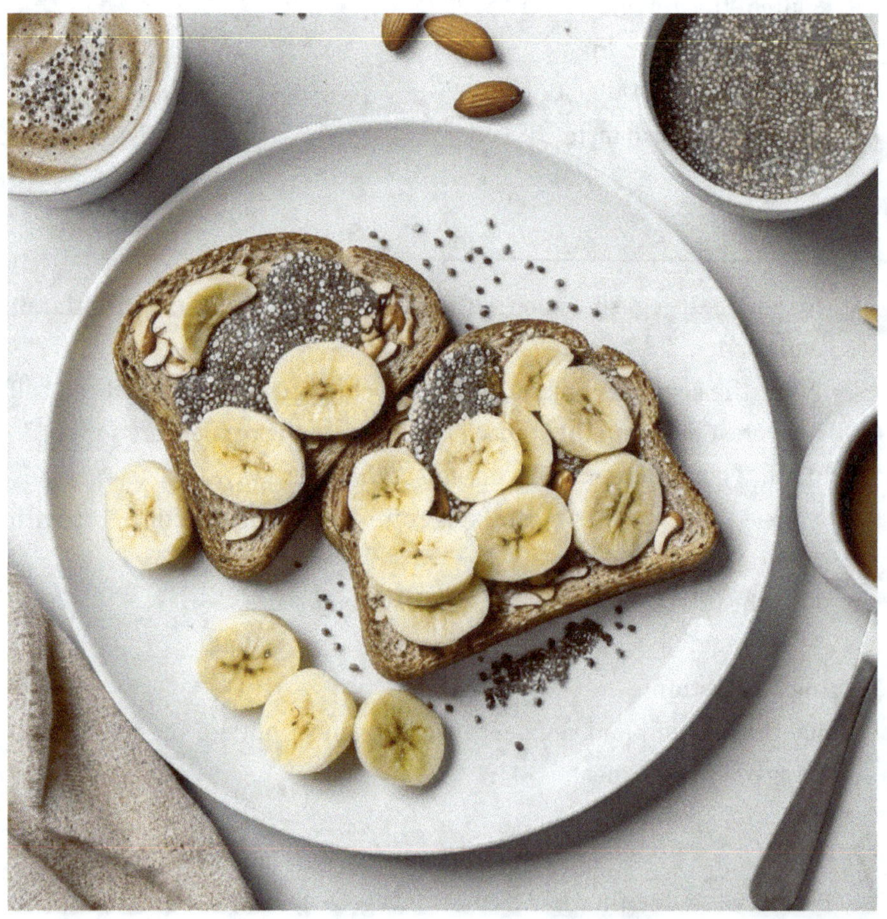

- **Yields:** 1 serving
- **Prep Time:** 2 minutes
- **Cook Time:** N/A
- **Total Time:** 2 minutes

Ingredients:

- 1 slice gluten-free bread
- 2 tablespoons nut butter (almond butter or peanut butter in moderation)
- ½ banana, sliced
- Chia seeds (optional, for topping)

Instructions:

1. Toast a slice of gluten-free bread.
2. Spread the nut butter of your choice onto the toast.
3. Top with sliced banana.
4. Sprinkle with chia seeds for added texture and nutrients (optional).

Serving Suggestion:

This is a simple and satisfying breakfast that requires minimal prep. Enjoy it as is, or pair it with a cup of lactose-free milk or tea for a more complete meal.

Notes:

- You can use any type of low-FODMAP nut butter you like, such as almond butter, cashew butter, or sunflower seed butter.
- If you don't have any gluten-free bread, you can use rice cakes or another low-FODMAP bread alternative.

* * *

Baked Apples with Cinnamon and Walnuts

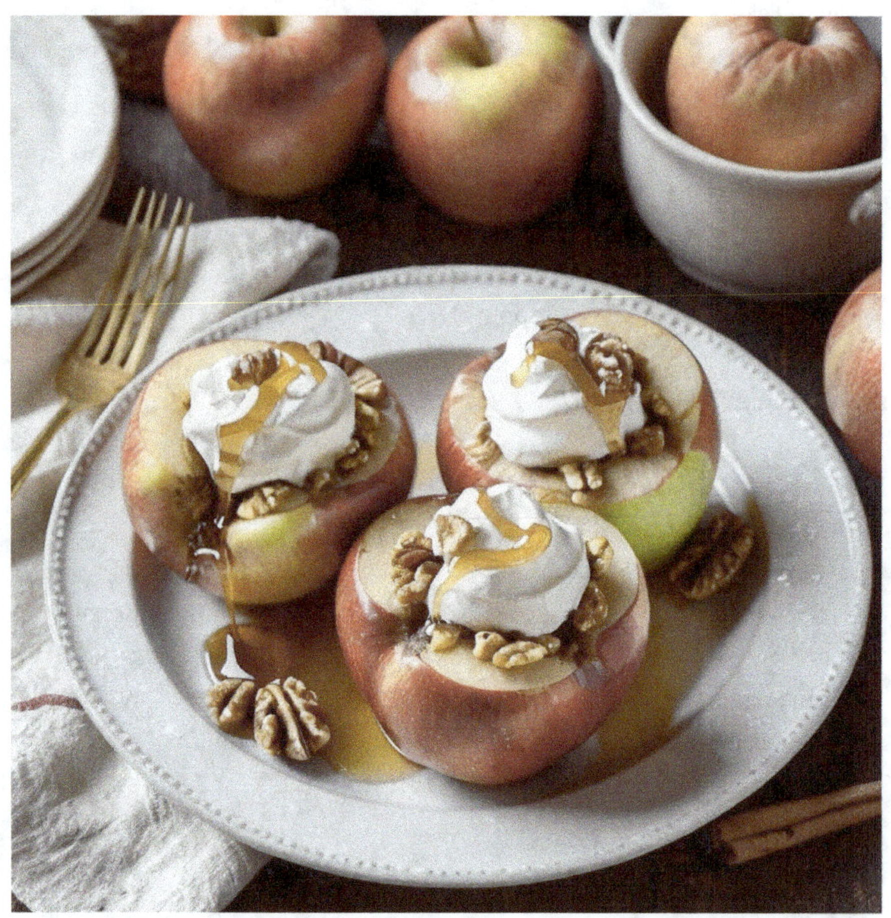

- **Yields:** 1 serving
- **Prep Time:** 10 minutes
- **Cook Time:** 20-25 minutes
- **Total Time:** 30-35 minutes

Ingredients:

- 1 apple (choose a low-FODMAP variety like Granny Smith or Gala)
- ½ teaspoon ground cinnamon
- ¼ cup chopped walnuts
- 1 tablespoon raisins (limited amount)
- 1 tablespoon lactose-free yogurt or milk alternative (optional)

Instructions:

1. Preheat oven to 375°F (190°C).
2. Core the apple, leaving the bottom intact.
3. In a small bowl, combine chopped walnuts, raisins, and cinnamon.
4. Stuff the apple core with the walnut mixture.
5. Place the apple in a baking dish and add a splash of water to the bottom of the dish to prevent burning.
6. Bake for 20-25 minutes, or until the apple is tender and the filling is bubbly.
7. Drizzle with a little lactose-free yogurt or milk alternative (optional) and serve warm.

Serving Suggestion:

Enjoy this warm and comforting baked apple for a delightful and healthy breakfast treat.

Notes:

- Be sure to choose a low-FODMAP variety of apple for this recipe.
- You can adjust the amount of raisins to your preference.
- Leftovers can be stored in an airtight container in the refrigerator for up to 2 days. Reheat gently in the microwave before serving.

With this variety of delicious and gut-friendly breakfast options, you can conquer your mornings and feel your best throughout the day. Remember, a healthy breakfast doesn't have to be bland or boring. The low-FODMAP world is full of flavor waiting to be explored!

Lunch and Salads

Lunchtime shouldn't be a battle with your IBS symptoms. This section is packed with 10 creative and satisfying low-FODMAP lunch and salad recipes designed to keep your gut happy and your taste buds singing.

* * *

Rainbow Veggie Power Bowl

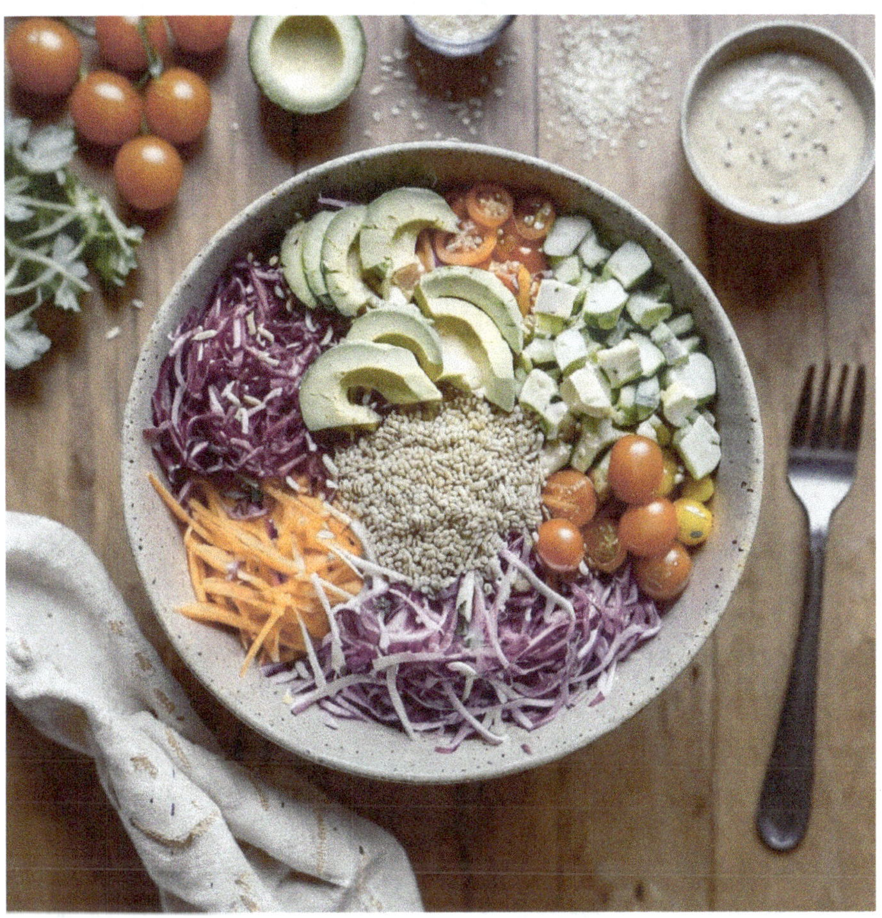

- **Yields:** 1 serving
- **Prep Time:** 15 minutes
- **Cook Time:** (depends on cooking time for quinoa and vegetables)
- **Total Time:** Prep time + Cook time for quinoa and vegetables

Ingredients:

- ½ cup cooked quinoa
- 1 cup roasted vegetables (combination of zucchini, bell peppers, cherry

tomatoes) - see roasting instructions below
- ½ cup grilled chicken breast, sliced (or other protein of choice)
- ¼ cup crumbled feta cheese (optional, in moderation)
- 2 tablespoons low-FODMAP vinaigrette dressing
- Fresh herbs (optional, for garnish): chopped parsley, cilantro, or chives

Instructions:

1. **For the roasted vegetables:** Preheat oven to 400°F (200°C). Chop zucchini, bell peppers, and cherry tomatoes into bite-sized pieces. Toss with a drizzle of olive oil and a sprinkle of salt and pepper. Spread the vegetables on a baking sheet and roast for 15-20 minutes, or until tender-crisp.
2. While the vegetables are roasting, cook your chosen protein according to your preferred method (grilling, baking, etc.). Slice the cooked protein into bite-sized pieces.
3. In a bowl, combine cooked quinoa, roasted vegetables, sliced protein, and crumbled feta cheese (if using).
4. Drizzle with your favorite low-FODMAP vinaigrette dressing and toss to coat.
5. Garnish with fresh chopped herbs (optional) and serve.

Serving Suggestion:
Enjoy this vibrant and nutrient-packed bowl for a satisfying and gut-friendly lunch.
Notes:

- You can customize the vegetables in this recipe based on your preferences and what's in season. Other low-FODMAP options include roasted eggplant, asparagus, or broccoli.
- Leftovers can be stored in an airtight container in the refrigerator for up to 3 days.

* * *

Mediterranean Tuna Salad Pita Pockets

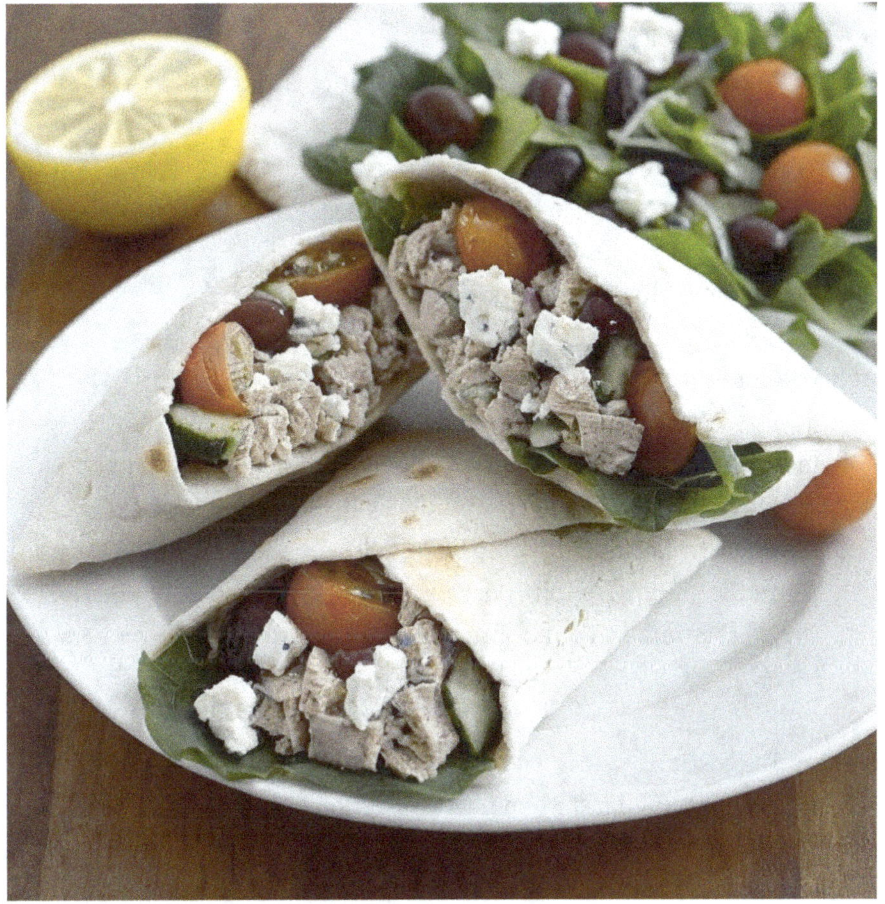

- **Yields:** 2 servings
- **Prep Time:** 10 minutes

- **Cook Time:** N/A
- **Total Time:** 10 minutes

Ingredients:

- 2 cans tuna in water (flaked)
- 1 chopped tomato
- ½ cucumber, diced
- ¼ cup crumbled feta cheese (optional, in moderation)
- ¼ cup chopped olives (kalamata or green)
- 1 tablespoon olive oil
- 1 tablespoon lemon juice
- Salt and pepper to taste
- 2 gluten-free pita pockets, warmed

Instructions:

1. In a bowl, combine flaked tuna, chopped tomato, diced cucumber, feta cheese (if using), chopped olives, olive oil, and lemon juice.
2. Season with salt and pepper to taste.
3. Warm the gluten-free pita pockets according to package instructions.
4. Divide the tuna salad mixture between the warmed pita pockets and serve.

Serving Suggestion:
Enjoy this protein-packed and flavorful option for a quick and easy lunch. Serve with a side salad for added greens.

Notes:

- You can adjust the amount of feta cheese to your preference.
- For a vegetarian option, substitute the tuna with cooked and crumbled lentils.

* * *

Creamy Lentil Soup with Gluten-Free Bread

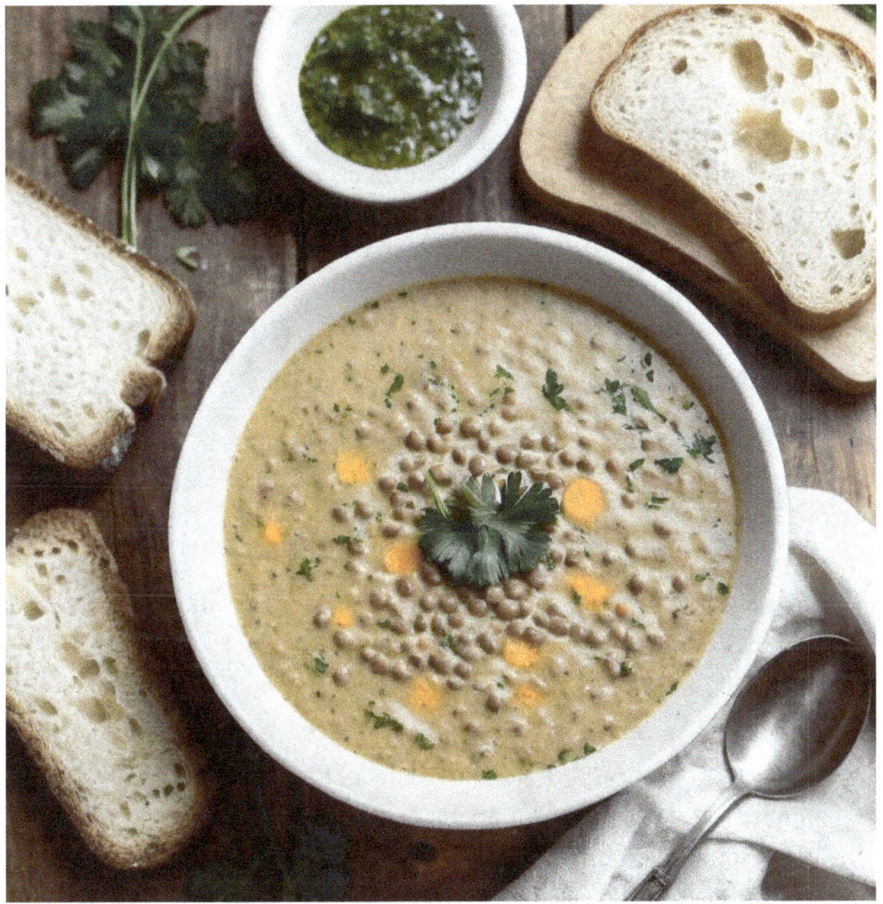

- **Yields:** 4 servings
- **Prep Time:** 10 minutes

- **Cook Time:** 30 minutes
- **Total Time:** 40 minutes

Ingredients:

- 1 tablespoon olive oil
- 1 onion, chopped
- 2 carrots, chopped
- 2 celery stalks, chopped
- 2 cloves garlic, minced
- 1 cup green lentils, rinsed
- 4 cups low-FODMAP vegetable broth
- 1 can (14.5 oz) diced tomatoes, undrained
- 1 teaspoon dried thyme
- ½ teaspoon dried rosemary
- Salt and pepper to taste
- 4 slices gluten-free bread, toasted (for serving)

Instructions:

1. Heat olive oil in a large pot over medium heat. Add onion, carrots, and celery. Sauté for 5 minutes, or until softened.
2. Add garlic and cook for an additional minute, until fragrant.
3. Stir in rinsed lentils, vegetable broth, diced tomatoes, thyme, and rosemary. Bring to a boil, then reduce heat and simmer for 20-25 minutes, or until the lentils are tender.
4. Using an immersion blender or a blender in batches, puree a portion of the soup to create a creamy texture (optional). Season with salt and pepper to taste.
5. Serve the soup hot with a slice of toasted gluten-free bread.

Serving Suggestion:
This hearty and comforting soup is perfect for a satisfying lunch. You can

add a sprinkle of chopped fresh herbs like parsley or chives for extra flavor.

Notes:

- You can adjust the thickness of the soup by adding more or less vegetable broth.
- Leftovers can be stored in an airtight container in the refrigerator for up to 3 days.

* * *

Chicken and Mango Salad with Coconut Curry Dressing

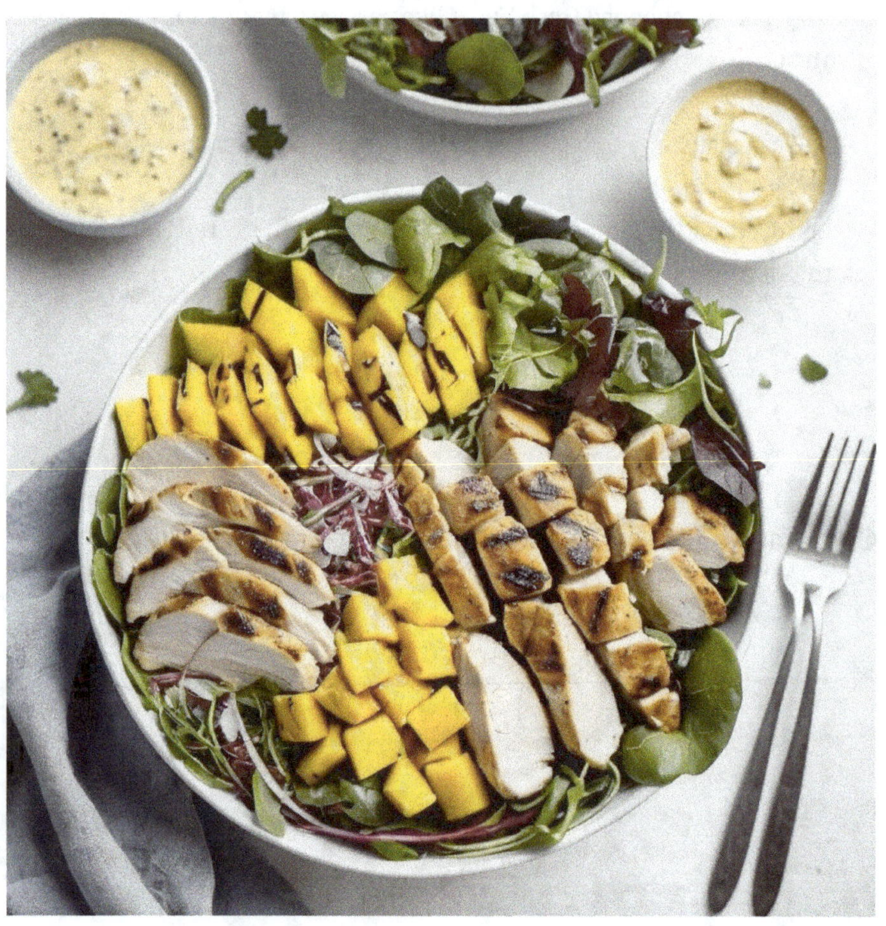

- **Yields:** 2 servings
- **Prep Time:** 15 minutes
- **Cook Time:** (depends on cooking time for chicken)
- **Total Time:** Prep time + Cook time for chicken

Ingredients:

- **For the Chicken:**
- 1 boneless, skinless chicken breast (or substitute with grilled shrimp or

tofu for a vegetarian option)
- Salt and pepper to taste
- **For the Salad:**
- 2 cups mixed greens (such as baby spinach, arugula, or a combination)
- 1 cooked chicken breast, sliced (or your chosen protein alternative)
- 1 ripe mango, diced
- ½ red onion, thinly sliced
- ¼ cup chopped fresh cilantro

For the Coconut Curry Dressing:

- ¼ cup canned coconut milk (full-fat for creamier texture)
- 1 tablespoon fresh lime juice
- 1 tablespoon low-FODMAP maple syrup (or use honey if tolerated)
- 1 teaspoon curry powder
- ½ teaspoon ground ginger
- Pinch of salt

Instructions:

1. **Cook the Chicken:** Season the chicken breast with salt and pepper. Grill, bake, or pan-cook the chicken according to your preferred method until cooked through. Let it cool slightly, then slice it into bite-sized pieces.
2. **Prepare the Dressing:** In a small bowl or jar with a lid, whisk together coconut milk, lime juice, maple syrup, curry powder, ground ginger, and salt. Shake well to combine if using a jar.
3. **Assemble the Salad:** In a large bowl, combine mixed greens, sliced chicken, diced mango, and red onion.
4. **Dress the Salad:** Drizzle the coconut curry dressing over the salad and toss gently to coat all ingredients.
5. **Serve and Enjoy:** Garnish with chopped fresh cilantro and serve immediately.

Serving Suggestion:

This flavorful salad is perfect for a light and satisfying lunch. Pair it with a side of gluten-free crackers or whole-wheat toast for a more complete meal.

Notes:

· Leftover salad can be stored in an airtight container in the refrigerator for up to 1 day. The dressing may separate, so give it a good shake before serving leftovers.
· Feel free to adjust the amount of curry powder to your spice preference.
· For a vegan option, use a plant-based yogurt alternative in the dressing instead of coconut milk.

* * *

Leftover Makeover Buddha Bowl

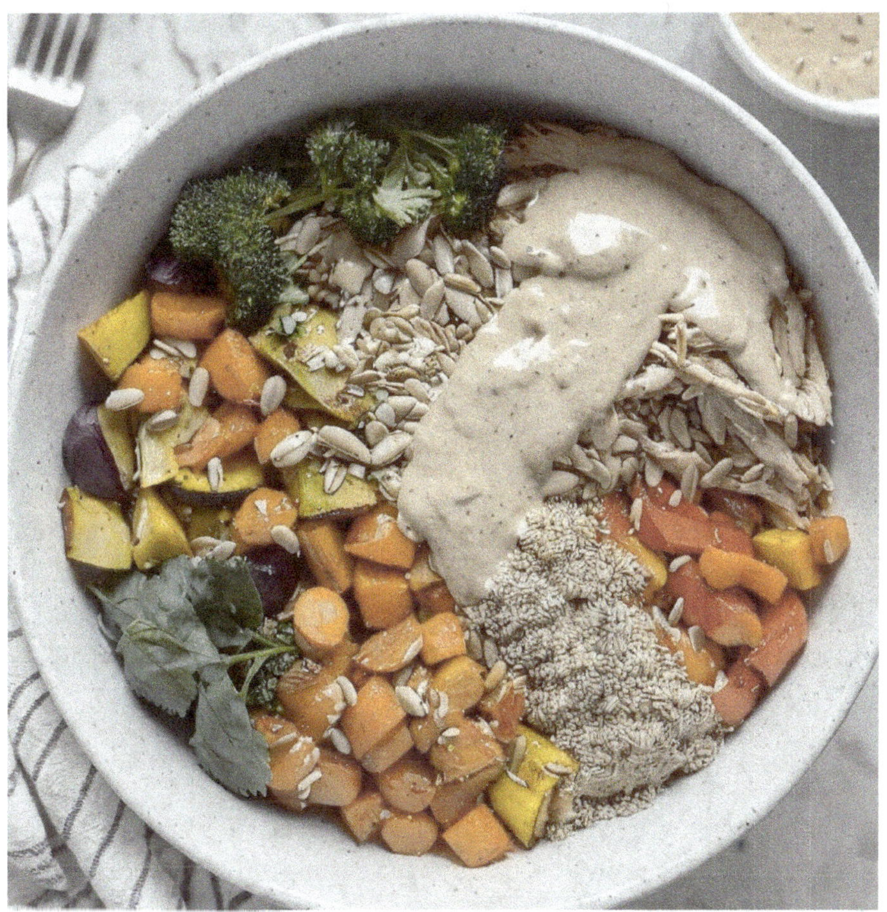

- **Yields:** 1 serving
- **Prep Time:** 10 minutes
- **Cook Time:** N/A
- **Total Time:** 10 minutes

Ingredients:

- 1 cup cooked quinoa, brown rice, or chopped vegetables (use leftover protein or roasted vegetables)

- ½ cup chopped low-FODMAP vegetables (cucumber, shredded carrots, cherry tomatoes)
- ¼ cup shredded cooked chicken or tofu (optional, use leftover protein)
- ¼ cup cooked lentils or chickpeas (optional)
- ¼ avocado, sliced
- 2 tablespoons chopped fresh herbs (parsley, cilantro, chives)
- Low-FODMAP vinaigrette dressing of your choice

Instructions:

1. In a bowl, combine your chosen base (cooked quinoa, brown rice, or chopped vegetables).
2. Add chopped low-FODMAP vegetables, cooked protein (chicken, tofu, lentils, or chickpeas), and sliced avocado.
3. Sprinkle with chopped fresh herbs.
4. Drizzle with your favorite low-FODMAP vinaigrette dressing and toss to coat.

Serving Suggestion:

This is a great way to use up leftover ingredients and create a delicious and nutritious lunch bowl. Get creative and customize it with your favorite low-FODMAP toppings!

Notes:

- Leftovers can be stored in an airtight container in the refrigerator for up to 2 days.

* * *

Spicy Thai Shrimp with Zoodles

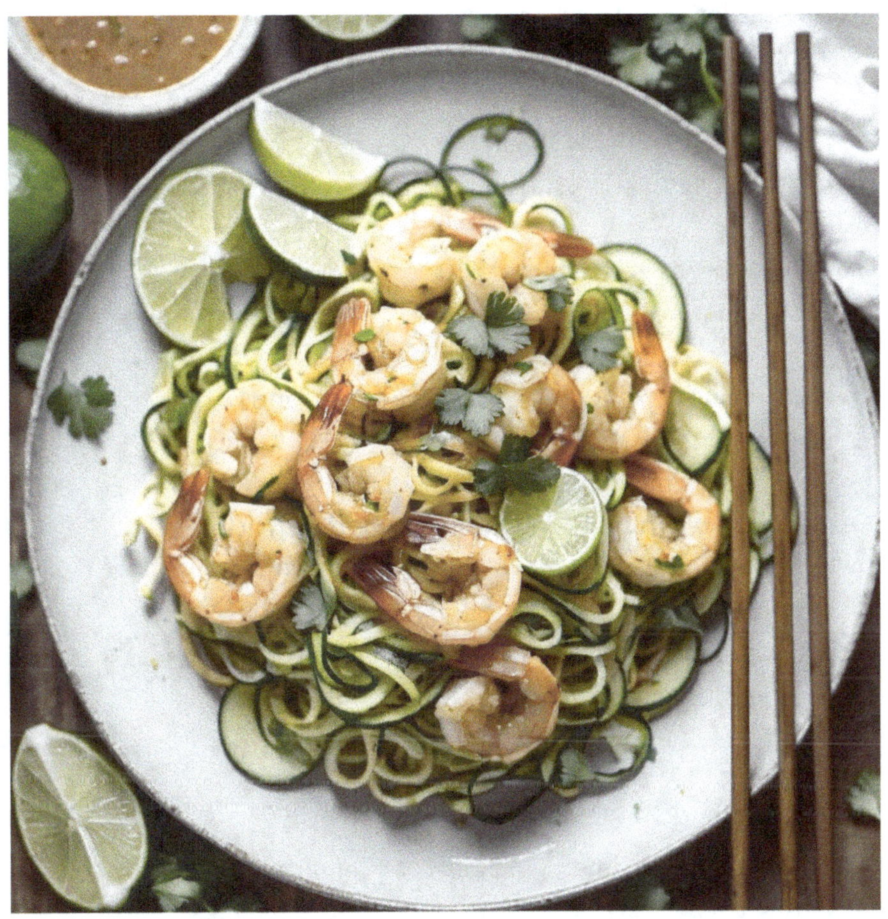

- **Yields:** 2 servings
- **Prep Time:** 10 minutes
- **Cook Time:** 10–12 minutes
- **Total Time:** 20–22 minutes

Ingredients:

- 1 pound fresh shrimp, peeled and deveined
- 1 tablespoon cornstarch (or arrowroot powder)
- 1 tablespoon olive oil
- 2 cloves garlic, minced
- 1 red bell pepper, thinly sliced
- ½ cup sugar snap peas, trimmed and halved (or sub with broccolini florets)
- ¼ cup chopped green onions
- **For the Sauce:**
- ¼ cup coconut milk
- 2 tablespoons low-FODMAP fish sauce (check label)
- 1 tablespoon lime juice
- 1 tablespoon brown sugar (or low-FODMAP maple syrup)
- 1 teaspoon red chili flakes (adjust for spice preference)
- ½ teaspoon ground ginger
- **For Serving:**
- 2 cups zucchini noodles (zoodles)
- Chopped fresh cilantro (optional)

Instructions:

1. **Marinate the Shrimp:** In a bowl, toss the shrimp with cornstarch (or arrowroot powder). Set aside to marinate for 5 minutes.
2. **Prepare the Sauce:** In a small bowl, whisk together coconut milk, fish sauce, lime juice, brown sugar (or maple syrup), red chili flakes, and ground ginger. Set aside.
3. **Cook the Zoodles:** Using a spiralizer or julienne peeler, create zucchini noodles (zoodles). Heat a large skillet or wok over medium-high heat. Add the zoodles and cook for 2-3 minutes, stirring occasionally, until slightly softened. Transfer the cooked zoodles to a bowl and set aside.
4. **Cook the Shrimp:** Heat the olive oil in the same skillet or wok over

medium-high heat. Add the shrimp and cook for 2-3 minutes per side, or until pink and opaque. Remove the cooked shrimp from the pan and set aside.

5. **Sauté the Vegetables:** Add the garlic, red bell pepper, and sugar snap peas (or broccolini) to the pan. Sauté for 2-3 minutes, or until the vegetables are slightly softened and crisp-tender.

6. **Combine and Simmer:** Pour the sauce mixture into the pan with the vegetables. Bring to a simmer and cook for 1-2 minutes, or until slightly thickened.

7. **Assemble and Serve:** Add the cooked shrimp and cooked zoodles back to the pan. Toss to coat everything in the sauce.

8. Serve immediately, garnished with chopped fresh cilantro (optional).

Serving Suggestion:

This light and flavorful dish is perfect for a warm day. Enjoy it as is, or serve it with a side of brown rice or quinoa for a more complete meal.

Notes:

- Be sure to check the label of your fish sauce to ensure it is low-FODMAP.
- You can adjust the amount of red chili flakes to your spice preference.
- Leftovers can be stored in an airtight container in the refrigerator for up to 1 day.

* * *

Turkey and Havarti Roll-Ups with Mustard Dip

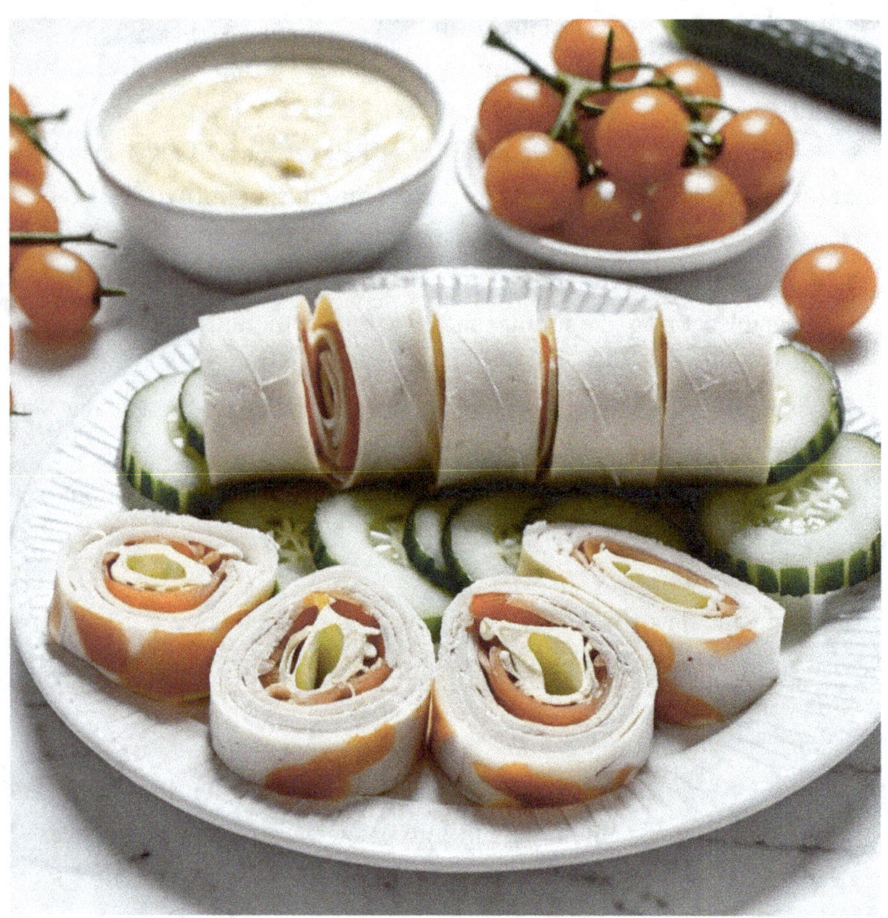

- **Yields:** 4 servings
- **Prep Time:** 15 minutes
- **Cook Time:** (depends on cooking time for turkey)
- **Total Time:** Prep time + Cook time for turkey

Ingredients:

- **For the Roll-Ups:**
- 8 slices gluten-free deli meat (turkey or chicken)

- 1 red bell pepper, thinly sliced
- 1 cup baby spinach
- ¼ cup crumbled Havarti cheese (optional, in moderation)
- Low-FODMAP mustard (Dijon or yellow mustard)
- **For the Mustard Dip:**
- ¼ cup lactose-free plain yogurt
- 2 tablespoons low-FODMAP mustard (Dijon or yellow mustard)
- 1 tablespoon chopped fresh chives

Instructions:

1. **Cook the Turkey:** If using raw turkey breast, cook it according to your preferred method (grilling, baking, etc.) until cooked through. Let it cool slightly and then slice it thinly. You can also use pre-sliced deli turkey or chicken breast.
2. **Prepare the Mustard Dip:** In a small bowl, whisk together lactose-free yogurt, mustard, and chopped fresh chives. Season with a pinch of salt and pepper to taste (optional, depending on the saltiness of your mustard).
3. **Assemble the Roll-Ups:** Spread a thin layer of mustard on each slice of gluten-free deli meat.
4. **Layer the Fillings:** Layer red bell pepper slices, baby spinach, and crumbled Havarti cheese (if using) on top of the mustard. Be sure to leave a small border at the edge to aid in rolling.
5. **Roll and Secure:** Roll up the deli meat tightly, enclosing the fillings. Secure the roll-up with a toothpick if desired, especially if using larger fillings.
6. **Serve and Enjoy:** Arrange the roll-ups on a platter and serve alongside the mustard dip for dipping.

Serving Suggestion:

These protein-packed and flavorful roll-ups are perfect for a quick and easy lunch or portable snack. Pair them with a side salad or sliced vegetables for a more complete meal.

Notes:

- You can adjust the amount of Havarti cheese to your preference and tolerance.
- Feel free to experiment with different low-FODMAP vegetables for the filling, such as shredded carrots, cucumber slices, or chopped olives.
- Leftover roll-ups can be stored in an airtight container in the refrigerator for up to 2 days.

* * *

Caprese Pasta Salad with Pesto

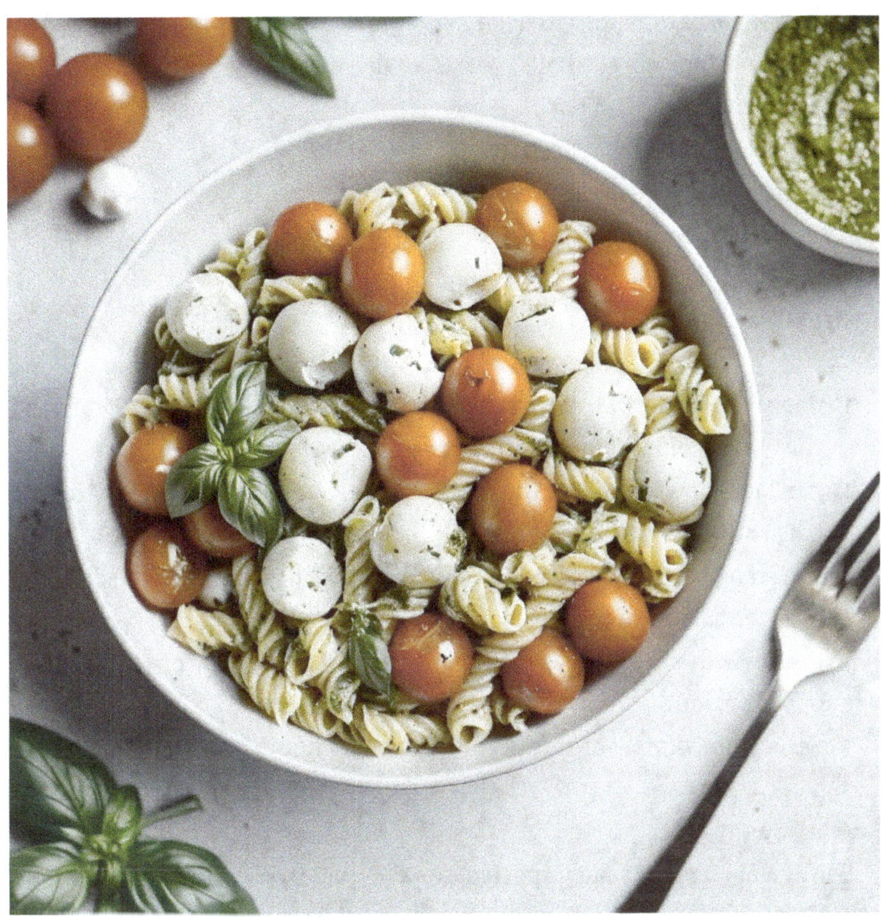

- **Yields:** 4 servings
- **Prep Time:** 15 minutes
- **Cook Time:** (depends on cooking time for pasta)
- **Total Time:** Prep time + Cook time for pasta

Ingredients:

- 8 ounces low-FODMAP pasta (such as gluten-free penne or brown rice pasta)

- 2 cups cherry tomatoes, halved
- 1 cup fresh mozzarella balls, pearls, or diced
- ½ cup chopped fresh basil
- ¼ cup low-FODMAP pesto
- 1 tablespoon olive oil
- Salt and pepper to taste

Instructions:

1. Cook the low-FODMAP pasta according to package directions. Drain and rinse with cold water to stop the cooking process.
2. In a large bowl, combine the cooked pasta, cherry tomatoes, mozzarella balls, and chopped fresh basil.
3. In a small bowl, whisk together the olive oil and pesto. Pour the dressing over the salad and toss to coat.
4. Season with salt and pepper to taste (optional, depending on the saltiness of your pesto).
5. Serve immediately or refrigerate for up to 2 hours before serving.

Serving Suggestion:

This flavorful pasta salad is perfect for a potluck or light lunch. For a more complete meal, serve it with a side of grilled chicken or fish.

Notes:

- Be sure to choose a low-FODMAP certified pesto or make your own using low-FODMAP ingredients.
- Leftovers can be stored in an airtight container in the refrigerator for up to 2 days. The flavors may meld even better overnight.

* * *

BLT Lettuce Wraps

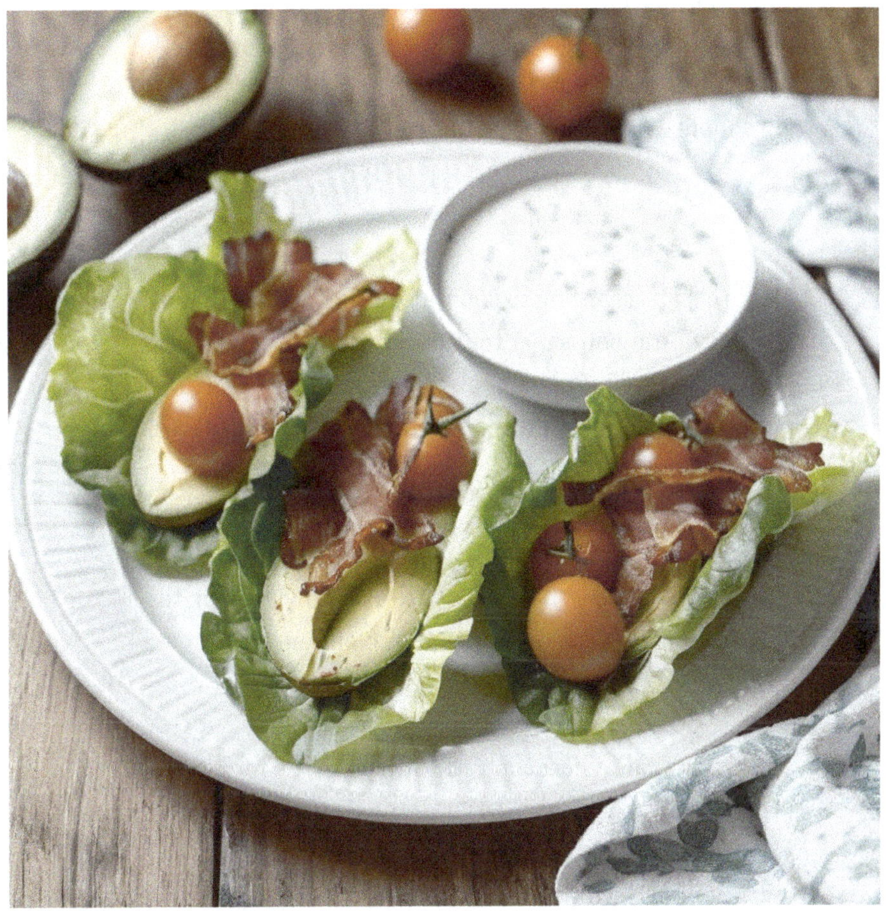

- **Yields:** 2 servings
- **Prep Time:** 10 minutes
- **Cook Time:** (depends on cooking method for bacon)
- **Total Time:** Prep time + Cook time for bacon

Ingredients:

- 4 large romaine lettuce leaves, washed and dried
- 4 slices crispy bacon
- 1 ripe tomato, sliced
- 2 tablespoons low-FODMAP mayonnaise
- ¼ cup chopped fresh chives

Instructions:

1. Cook the bacon according to your preferred method (frying, baking, etc.) until crispy. Drain on paper towels to remove excess grease.
2. Spread a thin layer of mayonnaise on each romaine lettuce leaf.
3. Top with sliced tomato, crumbled bacon, and chopped fresh chives.
4. Serve immediately.

Serving Suggestion:

These fun and flavorful lettuce wraps are a healthy twist on the classic BLT. They are perfect for a light lunch or low-carb option.

Notes:

- You can use avocado slices instead of mayonnaise for a dairy-free option.
- Feel free to add other low-FODMAP ingredients to your lettuce wraps, such as shredded carrots or chopped cucumber.
- Leftover cooked bacon can be stored in an airtight container in the refrigerator for up to 5 days.

* * *

Shrimp Scampi with Zucchini Noodles (Zoodles)

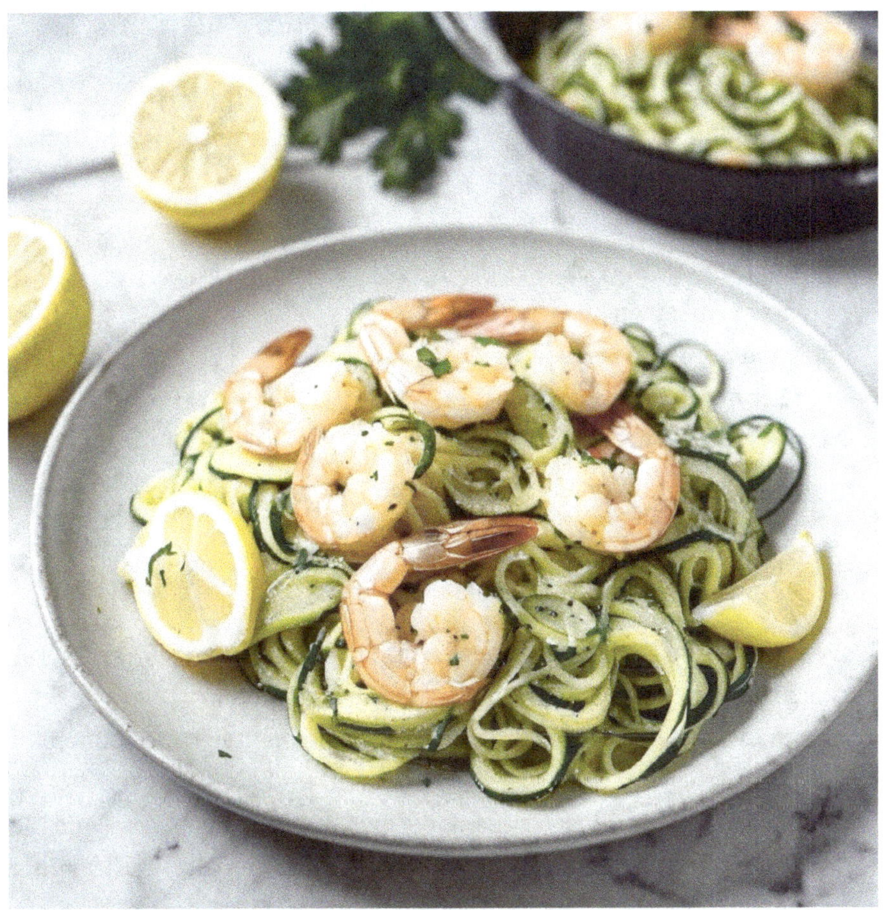

- **Yields:** 2 servings
- **Prep Time:** 10 minutes
- **Cook Time:** 10-12 minutes
- **Total Time:** 20-22 minutes

Ingredients:

- 1 pound fresh shrimp, peeled and deveined
- 1 tablespoon cornstarch (or arrowroot powder)
- 1 tablespoon olive oil
- 2 cloves garlic, minced
- ½ cup chopped cherry tomatoes
- ¼ cup chopped fresh parsley
- 2 tablespoons dry white wine (optional)
- ¼ cup low-FODMAP chicken broth
- 1 tablespoon lemon juice
- Salt and pepper to taste
- **For Serving:**
- 2 cups zucchini noodles (zoodles)
- Chopped fresh chives (optional)

Instructions:

1. **Marinate the Shrimp:** In a bowl, toss the shrimp with cornstarch (or arrowroot powder). Set aside to marinate for 5 minutes.
2. **Prepare the Zoodles:** Using a spiralizer or julienne peeler, create zucchini noodles (zoodles).
3. **Cook the Zoodles:** Heat a large skillet or wok over medium heat. Add the zoodles and cook for 2-3 minutes, stirring occasionally, until slightly softened. Transfer the cooked zoodles to a bowl and set aside.
4. **Cook the Shrimp:** Heat the olive oil in the same skillet or wok over medium-high heat. Add the shrimp and cook for 2-3 minutes per side, or until pink and opaque. Remove the cooked shrimp from the pan and set aside.
5. **Deglaze with Wine (Optional):** If using white wine, carefully pour it into the hot pan and scrape up any browned bits from the bottom. Let the wine simmer for a minute or two to allow the alcohol to cook off.
6. **Add Broth and Lemon Juice:** Add the low-FODMAP chicken broth and

lemon juice to the pan. Bring to a simmer and cook for 1-2 minutes, or until slightly reduced.

7. **Combine and Finish:** Add the cooked shrimp and chopped fresh parsley to the pan with the sauce. Toss to coat the shrimp in the sauce.
8. **Serve:** Plate the cooked zoodles and top with the shrimp scampi mixture. Garnish with chopped fresh chives (optional) and serve immediately.

Serving Suggestion:

This light and flavorful dish is perfect for a quick and easy weeknight meal. Enjoy it on its own or serve it with a side salad for a more complete meal.

Notes:

- If you choose to omit the white wine, you can add a splash of additional chicken broth or water to the pan in step 6.
- Leftovers can be stored in an airtight container in the refrigerator for up to 1 day. The zoodles may become softer upon reheating.

Dinner

One-Pan Salmon with Roasted Vegetables

A simple and flavorful sheet-pan meal with minimal cleanup.

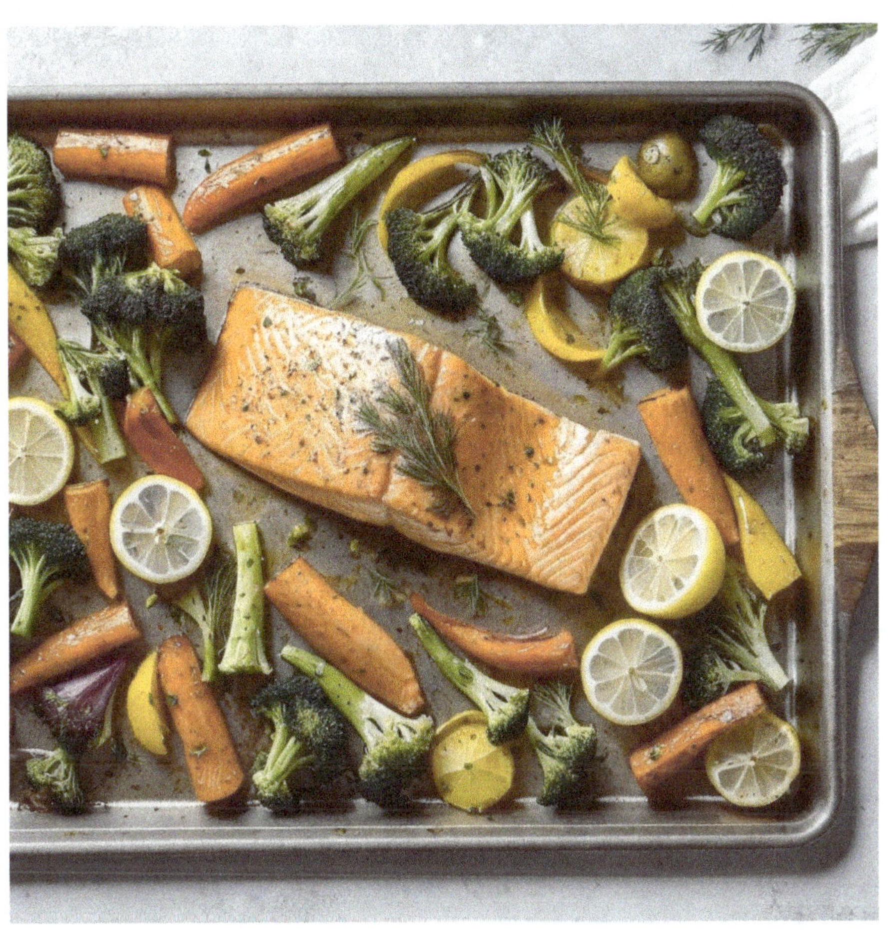

- **Yields:** 4 servings
- **Prep Time:** 10 minutes
- **Cook Time:** 20-25 minutes
- **Total Time:** 30-35 minutes

Ingredients:

- 4 salmon fillets (skin-on or off, depending on preference)

- 1 tablespoon olive oil
- Salt and pepper to taste
- 2 cups chopped low-FODMAP vegetables (broccoli florets, asparagus spears, cherry tomatoes)
- 1 tablespoon chopped fresh herbs (thyme, rosemary, parsley)
- 1 lemon, sliced (optional)

Instructions:

1. Preheat oven to 400°F (200°C).
2. Pat the salmon fillets dry with paper towels and season generously with salt and pepper.
3. In a large bowl, toss the chopped vegetables with olive oil, salt, pepper, and chopped herbs.
4. Spread the vegetables in a single layer on a rimmed baking sheet. Place the salmon fillets on top of the vegetables.
5. Arrange lemon slices around the salmon (optional).
6. Bake for 20-25 minutes, or until the salmon is cooked through and flakes easily with a fork. The vegetables should be tender-crisp.
7. Serve immediately.

Serving Suggestion:

Pair the salmon and roasted vegetables with a side of brown rice or quinoa for a complete meal.

Notes:

- You can substitute other low-FODMAP vegetables for the ones listed, such as green beans, zucchini, or bell peppers.
- Leftovers can be stored in an airtight container in the refrigerator for up to 3 days.

* * *

Creamy Vegetarian Chili with Cornbread

A satisfying and protein-packed chili perfect for a meatless Monday.

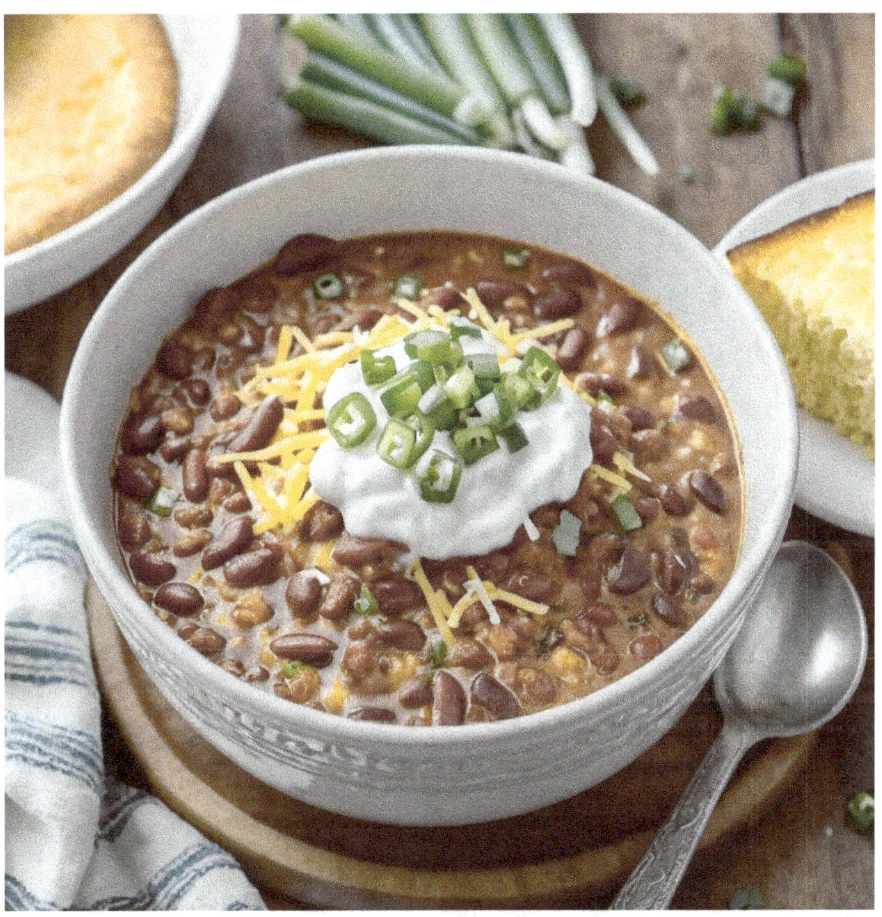

- **Yields:** 4-6 servings
- **Prep Time:** 15 minutes

- **Cook Time:** 30-35 minutes
- **Total Time:** 45-50 minutes

For the Chili:

- 1 tablespoon olive oil
- 1 onion, chopped
- 2 cloves garlic, minced
- 1 green bell pepper, chopped
- 1 red bell pepper, chopped
- 1 can (15 oz) diced tomatoes, undrained
- 1 can (15 oz) kidney beans, rinsed and drained
- 1 can (15 oz) black beans, rinsed and drained
- 4 cups low-FODMAP vegetable broth
- 1 tablespoon chili powder
- 1 teaspoon ground cumin
- ½ teaspoon smoked paprika
- Salt and pepper to taste
- **For the Cornbread (Optional):**
- Follow your favorite low-FODMAP cornbread recipe or use a gluten-free cornbread mix.

Instructions:

1. Heat olive oil in a large pot over medium heat. Add onion, garlic, bell peppers, and cook for 5 minutes, or until softened.
2. Stir in the diced tomatoes, kidney beans, black beans, vegetable broth, chili powder, cumin, smoked paprika, salt, and pepper.
3. Bring to a boil, then reduce heat and simmer for 20-25 minutes, or until the chili has thickened slightly.
4. While the chili simmers, prepare your cornbread according to package instructions (if using).
5. Serve the chili hot with a side of cornbread.

Serving Suggestion:

Top the chili with your favorite low-FODMAP toppings, such as chopped avocado, lactose-free sour cream, or chopped green onions.

Notes:

- You can adjust the amount of chili powder to your spice preference.
- Leftovers can be stored in an airtight container in the refrigerator for up to 3 days. The chili flavors may develop even better overnight.

* * *

Slow Cooker Low-FODMAP Beef Stew

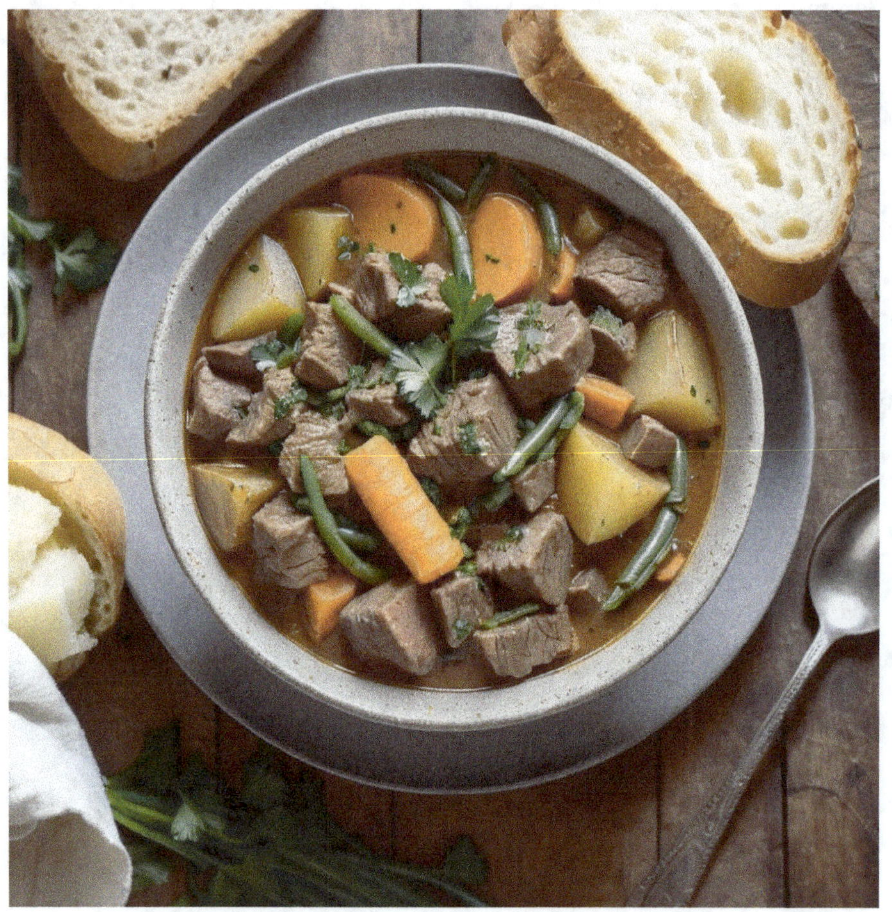

- **Yields:** 4-6 servings
- **Prep Time:** 15 minutes
- **Cook Time:** 6-8 hours on low, or 4-5 hours on high
- **Total Time:** Prep time + Cook time

Ingredients:

- 1 tablespoon garlic-infused olive oil (or other infused oil, like onion or shallot)

- 1 to 1 ½ pounds stew meat or boneless beef chuck, cut into 1-inch cubes
- 1 teaspoon Kosher salt, adjust to taste
- ½ teaspoon freshly ground black pepper, adjust to taste
- 2 cups baby red potatoes, quartered or in smaller pieces
- 1 ½ cups baby carrots, cut diagonally into 1/2-inch-thick slices
- 3 cups low-FODMAP beef broth (or chicken broth or vegan stock)
- 2 tablespoons tomato paste
- 1 tablespoon Worcestershire sauce (check label for low-FODMAP)
- 1 teaspoon dried thyme
- 1 teaspoon dried rosemary
- 1 teaspoon smoked paprika
- 2 bay leaves
- ¼ cup gluten-free low-FOPMAP all-purpose flour (or cornstarch slurry)

Instructions:

1. Heat the garlic-infused olive oil in a large skillet over medium heat. Season the beef with salt and pepper. Sear the beef in the skillet for 2-3 minutes per side, or until browned on all sides. This step is optional but adds depth of flavor.
2. Transfer the browned beef (or unseared beef if skipping that step) to a 6-quart slow cooker. Add the baby potatoes, baby carrots, beef broth, tomato paste, Worcestershire sauce, thyme, rosemary, paprika, and bay leaves. Stir to combine.
3. Cover the slow cooker and cook on low for 7-8 hours, or on high for 4-5 hours, or until the beef and vegetables are tender.
4. **Optional Thickening:** In a small bowl, whisk together ¼ cup of the stew broth with ¼ cup of gluten-free low-FODMAP flour (or cornstarch) to form a slurry. Stir the slurry into the slow cooker and cook for an additional 15 minutes on high, or until the stew reaches your desired thickness.
5. Remove the bay leaves before serving.
6. Serve the stew hot with crusty bread or a side salad.

Tips:

- Feel free to adjust the amount of smoked paprika to your spice preference.
- For a vegetarian option, substitute the beef with chickpeas or lentils. Add them to the slow cooker with the other vegetables in step 2.
- Leftovers can be stored in an airtight container in the refrigerator for up to 3 days or frozen for up to 3 months.

* * *

Thai Green Curry Chicken with Vegetables

A flavorful and aromatic curry packed with protein and veggies.

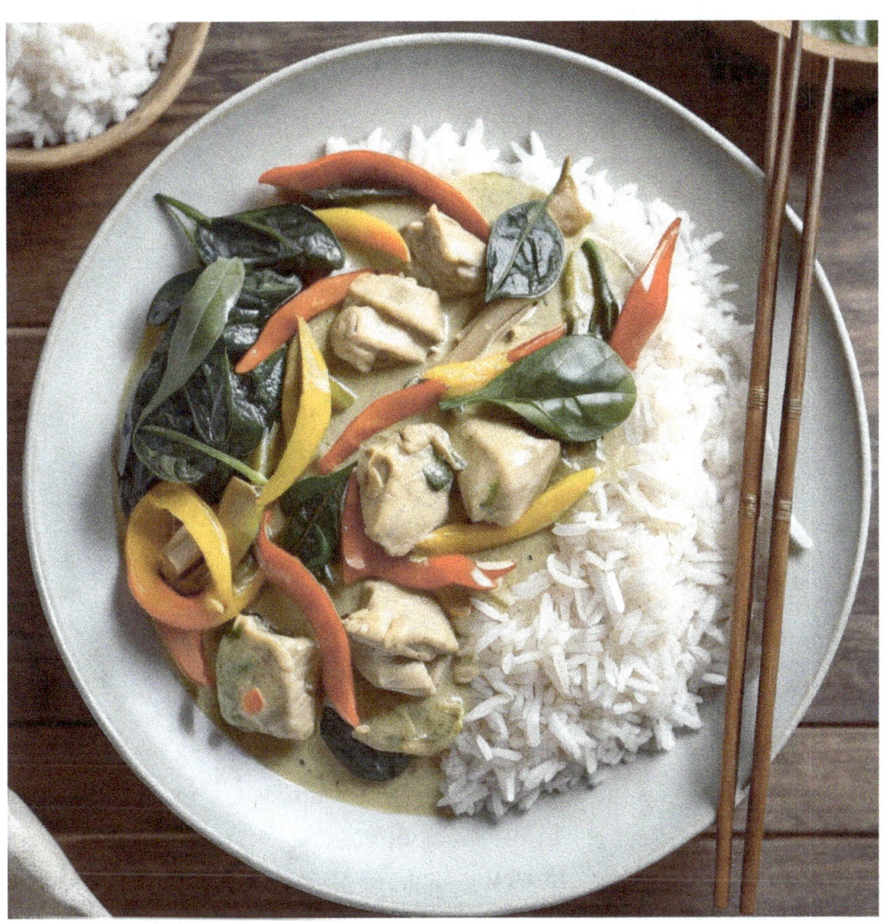

- **Yields:** 4 servings
- **Prep Time:** 15 minutes
- **Cook Time:** 20-25 minutes
- **Total Time:** 35-40 minutes

Ingredients:

- 1 tablespoon olive oil

- 1 pound boneless, skinless chicken breast, cut into bite-sized pieces
- 1 onion, chopped
- 2 cloves garlic, minced
- 1 red bell pepper, sliced
- 1 cup broccoli florets
- 1 green zucchini, sliced
- 1 can (13.5 oz) coconut milk (full-fat for creamier texture)
- 2 tablespoons green curry paste (check label for low-FODMAP)
- 1 tablespoon fish sauce (check label for low-FODMAP)
- 1 tablespoon brown sugar (or low-FODMAP maple syrup)
- 1 tablespoon lime juice
- Salt and pepper to taste
- Chopped fresh cilantro (optional, for garnish)
- Cooked rice or noodles (optional, for serving)

Instructions:

1. Heat olive oil in a large skillet or wok over medium heat. Add the chicken and cook for 5-7 minutes, or until browned and cooked through. Remove the chicken from the pan and set aside.
2. Add the onion and garlic to the pan and cook for 2-3 minutes, or until softened.
3. Stir in the red bell pepper, broccoli florets, and zucchini. Cook for 5-7 minutes, or until the vegetables are tender-crisp.
4. Add the coconut milk, green curry paste, fish sauce, brown sugar (or maple syrup), and lime juice to the pan. Bring to a simmer and cook for 2-3 minutes, or until slightly thickened.
5. Return the cooked chicken to the pan and stir to coat in the sauce.
6. Season with salt and pepper to taste.
7. Serve hot over cooked rice or noodles (optional) and garnish with chopped fresh cilantro (optional).

Serving Suggestion:

Pair this curry with a side of brown rice or quinoa for a complete meal. You can also serve it with gluten-free roti or naan bread for dipping.

Notes:

- The green curry paste can vary in spice level. Adjust the amount to your preference.
- Leftovers can be stored in an airtight container in the refrigerator for up to 3 days.

* * *

Sheet Pan Sausage and Peppers with Quinoa

A simple and colorful sheet-pan meal perfect for a busy weeknight.

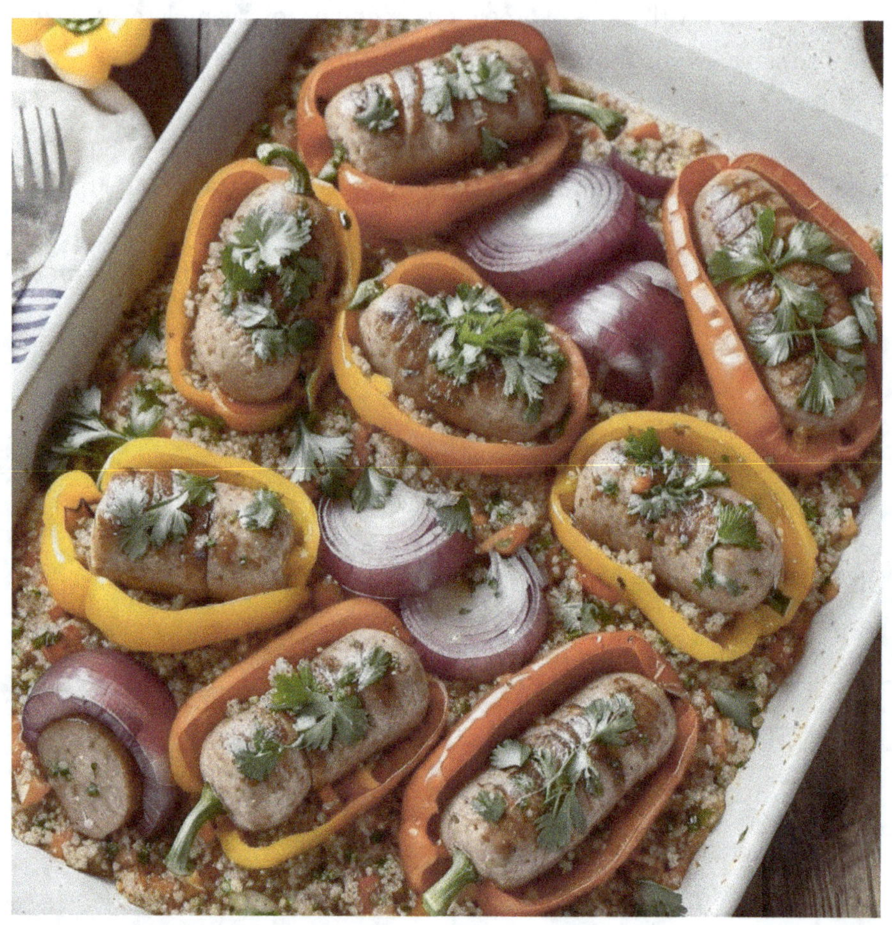

- **Yields:** 4 servings
- **Prep Time:** 15 minutes
- **Cook Time:** 20-25 minutes
- **Total Time:** 35-40 minutes

Ingredients:

- 1 tablespoon olive oil

- 1 pound Italian sausage links, casings removed (or substitute ground turkey or chicken sausage)
- 1 red bell pepper, sliced
- 1 yellow bell pepper, sliced
- 1 orange bell pepper, sliced
- 1 green bell pepper, sliced
- 1 red onion, sliced
- 1 cup quinoa, rinsed
- 1 ½ cups low-FODMAP vegetable broth
- ½ teaspoon dried thyme
- Salt and pepper to taste
- Chopped fresh parsley (optional, for garnish)

Instructions:

1. Preheat oven to 400°F (200°C).
2. In a large bowl, toss the Italian sausage, sliced bell peppers, red onion, olive oil, thyme, salt, and pepper.
3. Spread the sausage and vegetables in a single layer on a rimmed baking sheet.
4. In a separate bowl, combine the rinsed quinoa and vegetable broth. Pour the quinoa mixture over the sausage and vegetables on the baking sheet.
5. Bake for 20-25 minutes, or until the sausage is cooked through, the vegetables are tender-crisp, and the quinoa is cooked and fluffy.
6. Serve hot, garnished with chopped fresh parsley (optional).

Serving Suggestion:

This dish is delicious on its own, but you can also serve it with a side salad or roasted vegetables.

Notes:

- You can substitute other vegetables for the bell peppers, such as broccoli florets, cherry tomatoes, or asparagus spears.

- Leftovers can be stored in an airtight container in the refrigerator for up to 3 days.

* * *

Vegetarian Buddha Bowl with Tahini Dressing

A customizable and protein–packed bowl perfect for a satisfying and healthy meal.

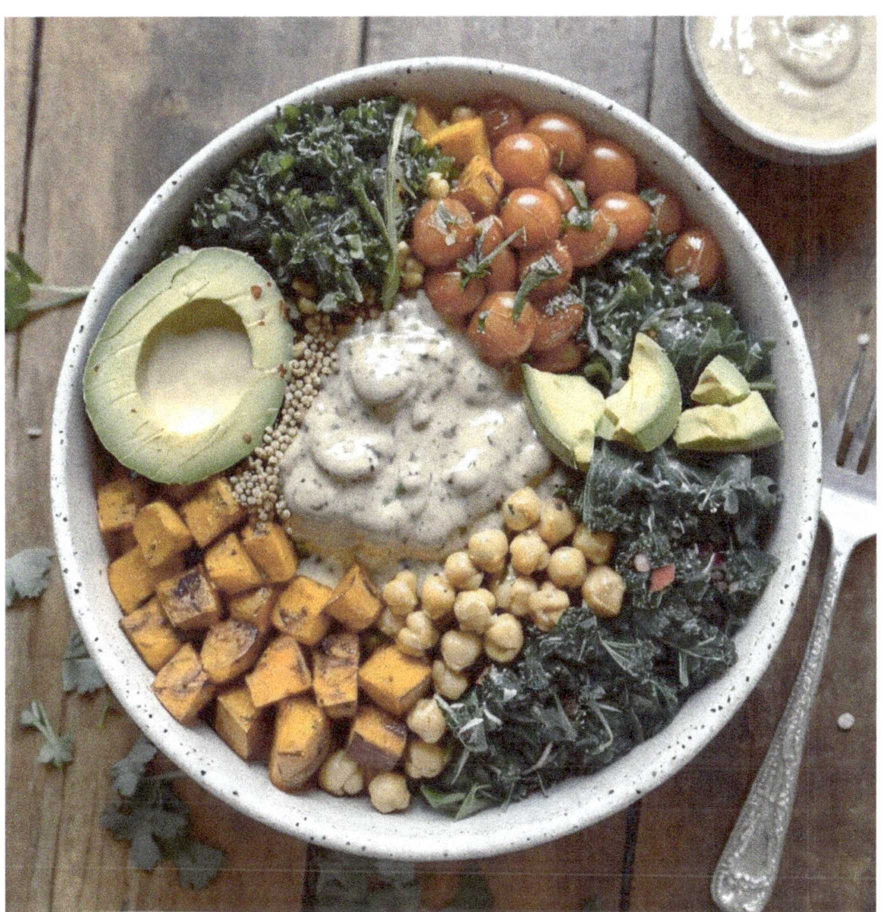

- **Yields:** 2 servings
- **Prep Time:** 15 minutes
- **Cook Time:** (depends on cooking time for individual ingredients)
- **Total Time:** Prep time + Cook time for individual ingredients

Ingredients:
For the Bowl:

- 1 cup cooked quinoa or brown rice
- ½ cup roasted chickpeas (or canned chickpeas, rinsed and drained)
- ½ cup roasted sweet potato cubes (or other roasted vegetables)
- ½ cup leafy greens (spinach, kale, etc.)
- ¼ cup shredded carrots
- ¼ cup crumbled feta cheese (optional)
- ¼ cup chopped avocado (optional)
- Sliced cherry tomatoes (optional)

For the Tahini Dressing:

- 2 tablespoons tahini
- 2 tablespoons lemon juice
- 1 tablespoon olive oil
- 1 tablespoon water
- 1 clove garlic, minced
- ½ teaspoon ground cumin
- Pinch of salt and pepper, to taste

Instructions:

1. **Prepare the Bowl Ingredients:** Cook the quinoa or brown rice according to package instructions. Roast the chickpeas and sweet potato cubes (or use other preferred roasted vegetables) until tender-crisp. Wash and chop any other desired raw vegetables.
2. **Assemble the Bowls:** Divide the cooked quinoa or brown rice between two bowls. Top with the roasted chickpeas, roasted vegetables, leafy greens, shredded carrots, crumbled feta cheese (if using), chopped avocado (if using), and sliced cherry tomatoes (if using).
3. **Make the Tahini Dressing:** In a small bowl, whisk together tahini, lemon juice, olive oil, water, minced garlic, ground cumin, salt, and pepper. Adjust seasonings to taste.
4. Drizzle the tahini dressing over each bowl and serve immediately.

Serving Suggestion:

This bowl is delicious on its own, but you can also serve it with a side of whole-wheat pita bread or crackers for dipping.

Notes:

- Feel free to customize the bowl with your favorite low-FODMAP ingredients.
- Leftovers can be stored in an airtight container in the refrigerator for up to 2 days.

* * *

One-Pot Creamy Tomato Chicken with Spinach

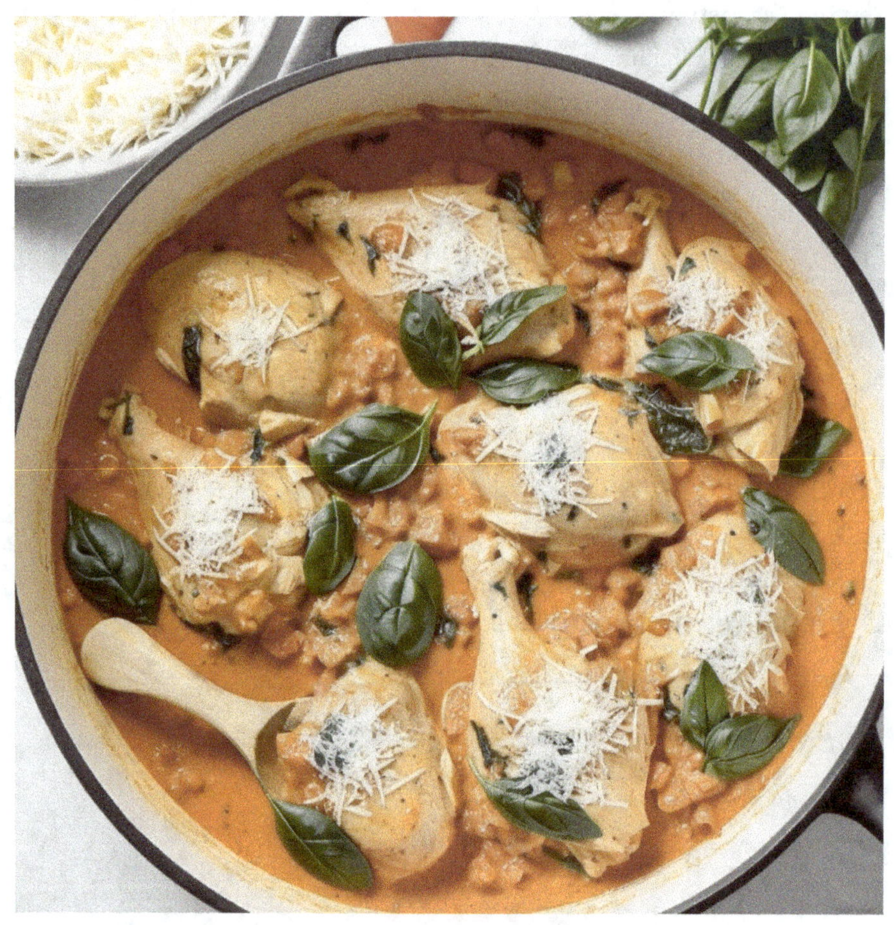

- **Yields:** 4 servings
- **Prep Time:** 10 minutes
- **Cook Time:** 20-25 minutes
- **Total Time:** 30-35 minutes

Ingredients:

- 1 tablespoon olive oil
- 1 pound boneless, skinless chicken breasts, cut into bite-sized pieces

- 1 onion, chopped
- 2 cloves garlic, minced
- 1 (14.5 oz) can diced tomatoes, undrained
- 1 cup low-FODMAP chicken broth
- ½ cup lactose-free heavy cream (or full-fat coconut milk)
- 2 tablespoons chopped fresh basil
- 1 tablespoon dried oregano
- ½ teaspoon salt
- ¼ teaspoon black pepper
- 4 cups baby spinach

Instructions:

1. Heat olive oil in a large pot or Dutch oven over medium heat. Add the chicken and cook for 5-7 minutes, or until browned on all sides.
2. Add the onion and garlic to the pot and cook for 2-3 minutes, or until softened.
3. Stir in the diced tomatoes (with their juices), chicken broth, heavy cream (or coconut milk), basil, oregano, salt, and pepper.
4. Bring to a simmer and cook for 10-12 minutes, or until the chicken is cooked through.
5. Stir in the baby spinach and cook for 1-2 minutes, or until wilted.
6. Serve immediately over cooked rice or pasta (optional).

Serving Suggestion:

Pair this creamy tomato chicken with a side of brown rice or quinoa for a complete meal. You can also serve it with crusty bread for dipping.

Notes:

- You can adjust the amount of dried oregano to your preference.
- Leftovers can be stored in an airtight container in the refrigerator for up to 3 days.

* * *

Lemon Garlic Shrimp with Zucchini Noodles (Zoodles)

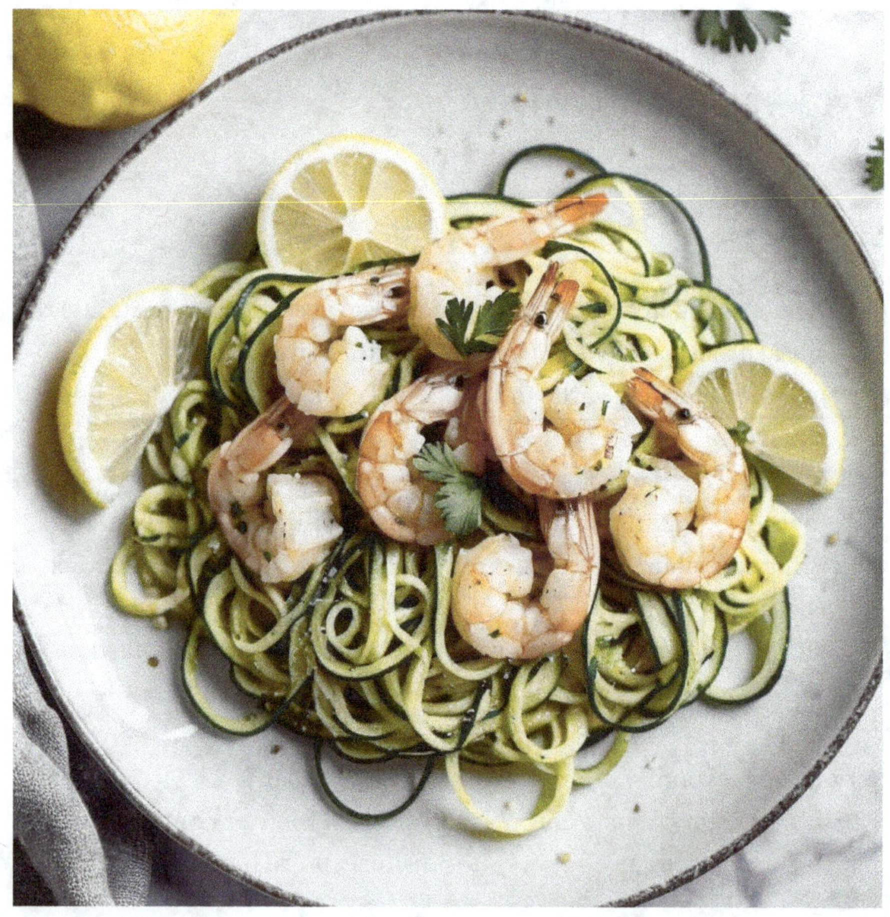

- **Yields:** 2 servings
- **Prep Time:** 10 minutes

- **Cook Time:** 10-12 minutes
- **Total Time:** 20-22 minutes

Ingredients:

- 1 pound fresh shrimp, peeled and deveined
- 1 tablespoon cornstarch (or arrowroot powder)
- 1 tablespoon olive oil
- 2 cloves garlic, minced
- ½ cup chopped cherry tomatoes
- ¼ cup chopped fresh parsley
- 2 tablespoons dry white wine (optional)
- ¼ cup low-FODMAP chicken broth
- 1 tablespoon lemon juice
- Salt and pepper to taste
- **For Serving:**
- 2 cups zucchini noodles (zoodles)
- Chopped fresh chives (optional)

Instructions:

1. **Marinate the Shrimp:** In a bowl, toss the shrimp with cornstarch (or arrowroot powder). Set aside to marinate for 5 minutes.
2. **Prepare the Zoodles:** Using a spiralizer or julienne peeler, create zucchini noodles (zoodles).
3. **Cook the Zoodles:** Heat a large skillet or wok over medium heat. Add the zoodles and cook for 2-3 minutes, stirring occasionally, until slightly softened. Transfer the cooked zoodles to a bowl and set aside.
4. **Cook the Shrimp:** Heat the olive oil in the same skillet or wok over medium-high heat. Add the shrimp and cook for 2-3 minutes per side, or until pink and opaque. Remove the cooked shrimp from the pan and set aside.
5. **Deglaze with Wine (Optional):** If using white wine, carefully pour it into

the hot pan and scrape up any browned bits from the bottom. Let the wine simmer for a minute or two to allow the alcohol to cook off.

6. **Add Broth and Lemon Juice:** Add the low-FODMAP chicken broth and lemon juice to the pan. Bring to a simmer and cook for 1-2 minutes, or until slightly reduced.

7. **Combine and Finish:** Add the cooked shrimp and chopped fresh parsley to the pan with the sauce. Toss to coat the shrimp in the sauce.

8. **Serve:** Plate the cooked zoodles and top with the shrimp scampi mixture. Garnish with chopped fresh chives (optional) and serve immediately.

Serving Suggestion:

This light and flavorful dish is perfect for a quick and easy weeknight meal. Enjoy it on its own or serve it with a side salad for a more complete meal.

Notes:

- If you choose to omit the white wine, you can add a splash of additional chicken broth or water to the pan in step 6.
- Leftovers can be stored in an airtight container in the refrigerator for up to 1 day. The zoodles may become softer upon reheating.

* * *

Chicken Fajitas with Spicy Mango Salsa:

A fun and flavorful twist on classic fajitas, perfect for a crowd or a fun weeknight dinner.

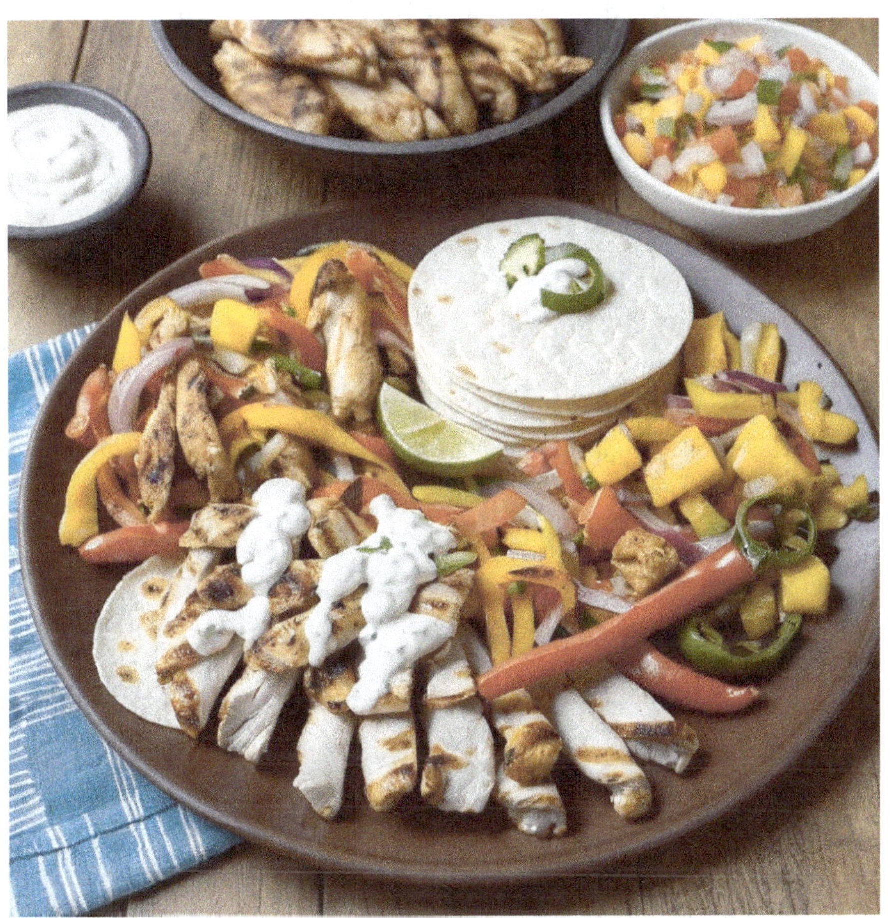

- **Yields:** 4 servings
- **Prep Time:** 15 minutes
- **Cook Time:** 20-25 minutes
- **Total Time:** 35-40 minutes

Ingredients:

- **For the Chicken Fajitas:**

- 1 pound boneless, skinless chicken breasts, thinly sliced
- 1 tablespoon olive oil
- 1 onion, sliced
- 1 green bell pepper, sliced
- 1 red bell pepper, sliced
- 1 teaspoon chili powder
- 1 teaspoon smoked paprika
- ½ teaspoon ground cumin
- ½ teaspoon garlic powder
- Salt and pepper to taste
- **For the Spicy Mango Salsa:**
- 1 ripe mango, peeled and diced
- 1 red bell pepper, seeded and diced
- 1/4 cup chopped red onion
- 1 jalapeño pepper, seeded and minced (optional, adjust for spice prefer-ence)
- 1 tablespoon chopped fresh cilantro
- 1 tablespoon lime juice
- Salt and pepper to taste
- **For Serving:**
- 4 low-carb tortillas (corn or wheat)
- Guacamole (optional)
- Sour cream (optional)
- Chopped lettuce (optional)

Instructions:

1. **Make the Spicy Mango Salsa:** In a bowl, combine diced mango, red bell pepper, red onion, jalapeño (if using), cilantro, lime juice, salt, and pepper. Stir well and set aside.

2. **Marinate the Chicken (Optional):** In a bowl, toss the sliced chicken breasts with olive oil, chili powder, smoked paprika, cumin, garlic powder, salt, and pepper. Marinate for 15 minutes (or up to 30 minutes)

for extra flavor, but this step is optional.

3. **Cook the Chicken Fajitas:** Heat a large skillet or grill pan over medium-high heat. Add the sliced onion and bell peppers and cook for 5-7 minutes, or until softened. Remove the vegetables from the pan and set aside.

4. If you marinated the chicken, add it to the hot pan and cook for 5-7 minutes per side, or until cooked through. If not marinating, simply cook the chicken until browned and cooked through.

5. **Warm the Tortillas:** While the chicken cooks, warm the tortillas according to package instructions.

6. **Assemble the Fajitas:** Serve the cooked chicken and fajita vegetables on warmed tortillas. Top with desired toppings like spicy mango salsa, guacamole, sour cream, and chopped lettuce.

Serving Suggestion:

These fajitas are delicious on their own or served with a side of Spanish rice or black beans.

Notes:

- You can adjust the amount of jalapeño pepper in the salsa to your spice preference.
- Leftover chicken fajita filling can be stored in an airtight container in the refrigerator for up to 3 days.

* * *

Turkey Burgers with Roasted Sweet Potato Fries

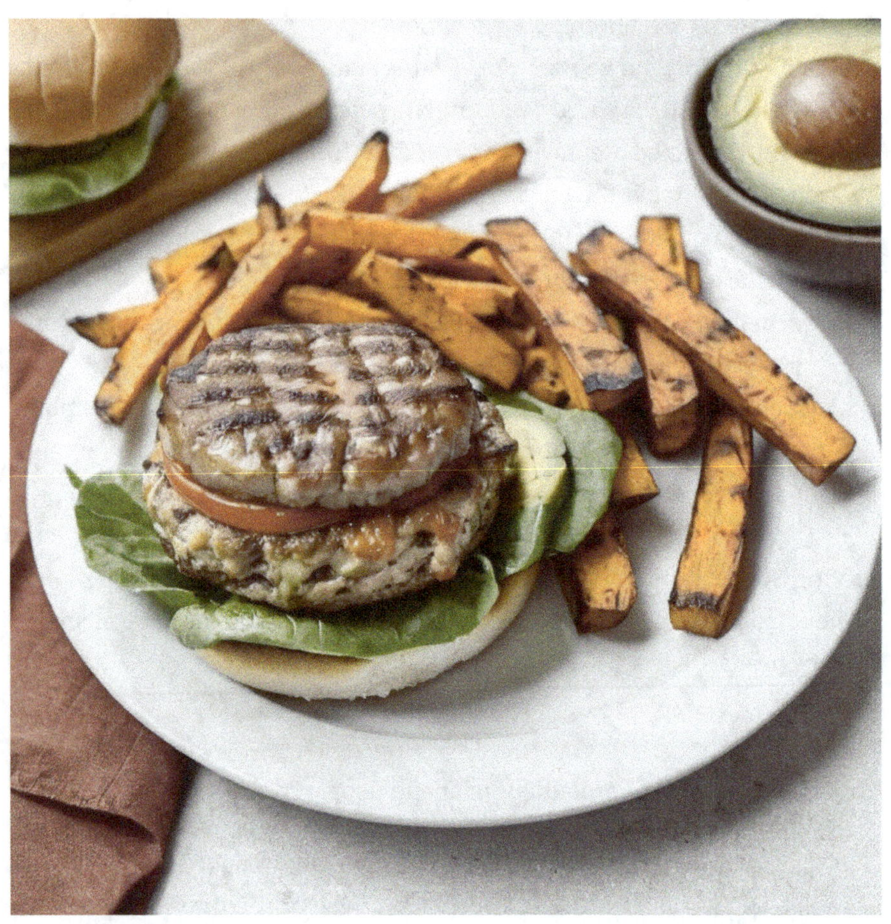

- **Yields:** 4 servings
- **Prep Time:** 15 minutes
- **Cook Time:** 20-25 minutes
- **Total Time:** 35-40 minutes

Ingredients:

For the Turkey Burgers:

- 1 pound ground turkey

- ½ cup chopped onion
- ¼ cup chopped fresh parsley
- 1 tablespoon Worcestershire sauce (check label for low-FODMAP)
- 1 egg, beaten
- ½ teaspoon dried thyme
- Salt and pepper to taste

For the Roasted Sweet Potato Fries:

- 2 large sweet potatoes, peeled and cut into wedges
- 1 tablespoon olive oil
- ½ teaspoon smoked paprika
- ½ teaspoon garlic powder
- Salt and pepper to taste

Instructions:

1. **Preheat Oven to 425°F (220°C):** Line a baking sheet with parchment paper.
2. **Prepare the Sweet Potato Fries:** In a large bowl, toss the sweet potato wedges with olive oil, smoked paprika, garlic powder, salt, and pepper. Spread the seasoned sweet potato wedges on the prepared baking sheet.
3. **Bake the Sweet Potato Fries:** Bake the sweet potato fries for 20-25 minutes, or until tender and golden brown, flipping halfway through baking.
4. **Make the Turkey Burgers:** While the sweet potato fries bake, in a large bowl, combine ground turkey, chopped onion, chopped parsley, Worcestershire sauce, beaten egg, dried thyme, salt, and pepper. Mix gently with your hands until just combined. Avoid overmixing.
5. **Form the Turkey Patties:** Divide the turkey mixture into four equal portions. Shape each portion into a patty that is slightly wider than your hamburger bun.
6. **Cook the Turkey Burgers:** Heat a large skillet or grill pan over medium

heat. Add the formed turkey patties and cook for 4–5 minutes per side, or until cooked through.

7. **Assemble and Serve:** Toast your hamburger buns according to package instructions (optional). Serve the cooked turkey burgers on toasted buns with your favorite burger toppings and a side of the roasted sweet potato fries.

Serving Suggestion:

Enjoy these healthier turkey burgers with classic hamburger toppings like lettuce, tomato, onion, pickles, ketchup, and mustard. You can also add a slice of low-FODMAP cheese (optional) for an extra layer of flavor.

Notes:

- You can adjust the seasonings in the turkey burgers to your preference.
- Leftover cooked burgers can be stored in an airtight container in the refrigerator for up to 3 days.

* * *

Black Bean Burgers with Chipotle Mayo

A delicious and protein-packed vegetarian burger option perfect for grilling or pan-frying.

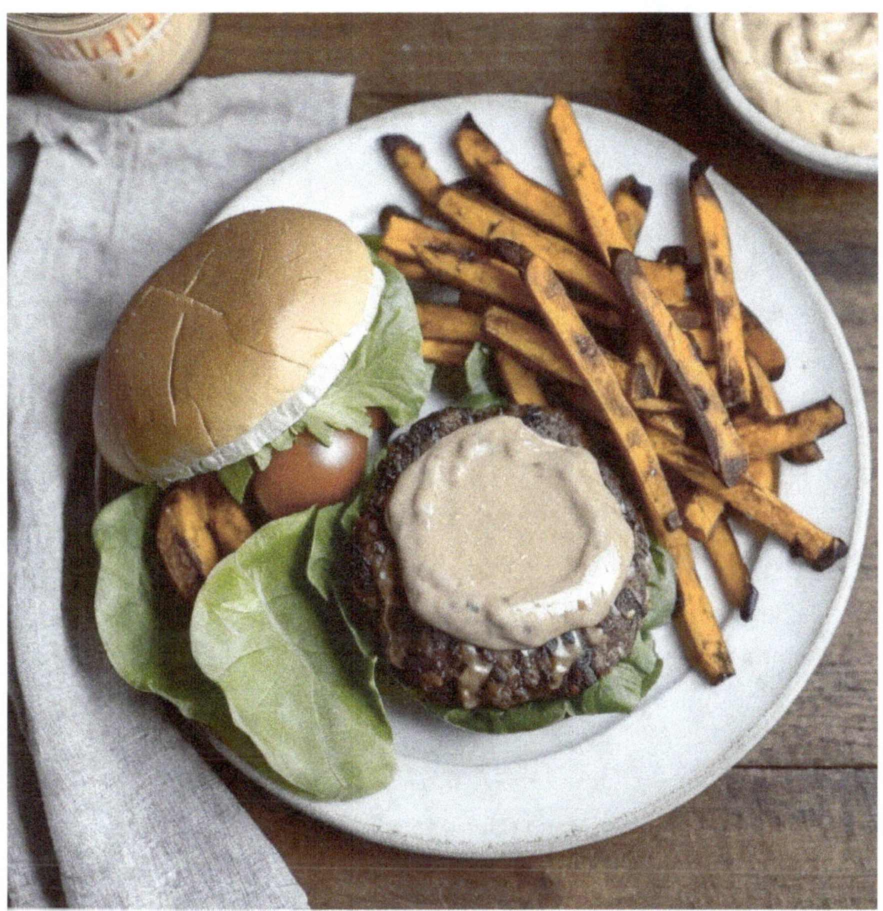

- **Yields:** 4 servings
- **Prep Time:** 15 minutes
- **Cook Time:** 10-12 minutes
- **Total Time:** 25-27 minutes

Ingredients:

- **For the Black Bean Burgers:**

- 1 (15 oz) can black beans, rinsed and drained
- 1 cup cooked brown rice
- ½ cup rolled oats
- ¼ cup chopped red onion
- 2 tablespoons chopped fresh cilantro
- 1 tablespoon olive oil
- 1 tablespoon chipotle powder (adjust for spice preference)
- 1 teaspoon ground cumin
- ½ teaspoon smoked paprika
- Salt and pepper to taste
- **For the Chipotle Mayo (Optional):**
- ½ cup mayonnaise
- 1 tablespoon canned chipotle peppers in adobo sauce, minced (adjust for spice preference)
- 1 tablespoon lime juice
- Salt and pepper to taste

Instructions:

1. **Make the Chipotle Mayo (Optional):** In a small bowl, combine mayonnaise, minced chipotle peppers in adobo sauce, lime juice, salt, and pepper. Stir well and set aside.

2. **Prepare the Black Bean Burger Mixture:** In a large bowl, mash the drained black beans with a fork or potato masher until slightly chunky. Do not completely puree the beans.

3. Add the cooked brown rice, rolled oats, chopped red onion, chopped cilantro, olive oil, chipotle powder, ground cumin, smoked paprika, salt, and pepper to the mashed black beans. Mix well to combine.

4. **Form the Black Bean Patties:** Divide the black bean mixture into four equal portions. Shape each portion into a patty that is slightly wider than your hamburger bun.

5. **Cook the Black Bean Burgers:** Heat a large skillet or grill pan over medium heat. Add the formed black bean patties and cook for 5-6

minutes per side, or until heated through and slightly browned.

6. **Assemble and Serve:** Toast your hamburger buns according to package instructions (optional). Serve the cooked black bean burgers on toasted buns with your favorite burger toppings and a dollop of chipotle mayo (optional).

Serving Suggestion:

These black bean burgers are delicious with classic burger toppings like lettuce, tomato, onion, pickles, ketchup, and mustard. You can also add a slice of low-FODMAP cheese (optional) for an extra layer of flavor.

Notes:

- You can adjust the amount of chipotle powder in the burgers and chipotle mayo to your spice preference.
- Leftover cooked burgers can be stored in an airtight container in the refrigerator for up to 3 days.

III

Living with Low-FODMAP

Dining Out on a Low-FODMAP Diet

Living with IBS can make navigating restaurant menus a challenge. But fear not! With a little planning and communication, you can still enjoy delicious meals out while staying true to your low-FODMAP journey. This chapter will equip you with tips and strategies for conquering restaurant dining with IBS.

Low-FODMAP Snacks and Treats

Sticking to a low-FODMAP diet doesn't mean sacrificing delicious snacks and treats! This chapter offers a variety of healthy and satisfying options to keep you energized and happy throughout the day.

* * *

Fruit and Nut Skewers

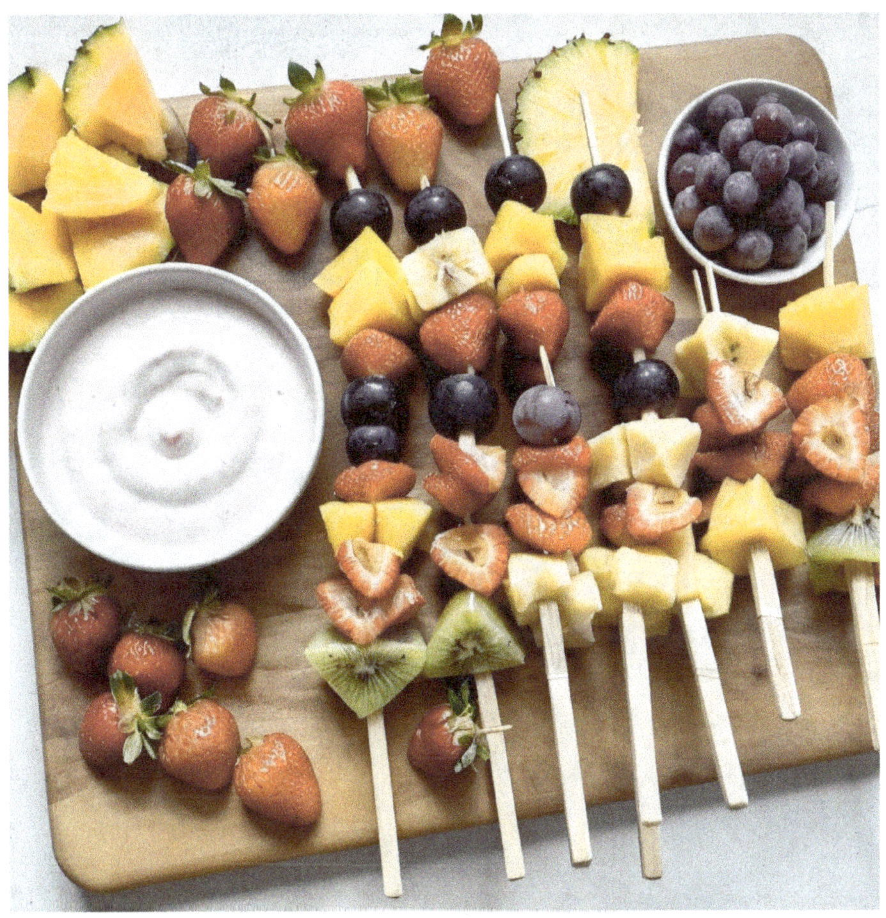

- **Yields:** 2-3 servings
- **Prep Time:** 5 minutes
- **Total Time:** 5 minutes

Ingredients:

- 1 cup mixed low-FODMAP fruits (strawberries, blueberries, grapes)
- ½ cup chopped nuts (almonds, walnuts, pecans)

Instructions:

1. Wash and dry the fruits.
2. Thread the fruits onto skewers, alternating colors and textures for visual appeal (optional).
3. Store leftover skewers in an airtight container in the refrigerator for up to 2 days.

Serving Suggestion:

Pair the fruit and nut skewers with a small container of low–FODMAP yogurt for dipping if desired.

* * *

Edamame with Chili and Lime

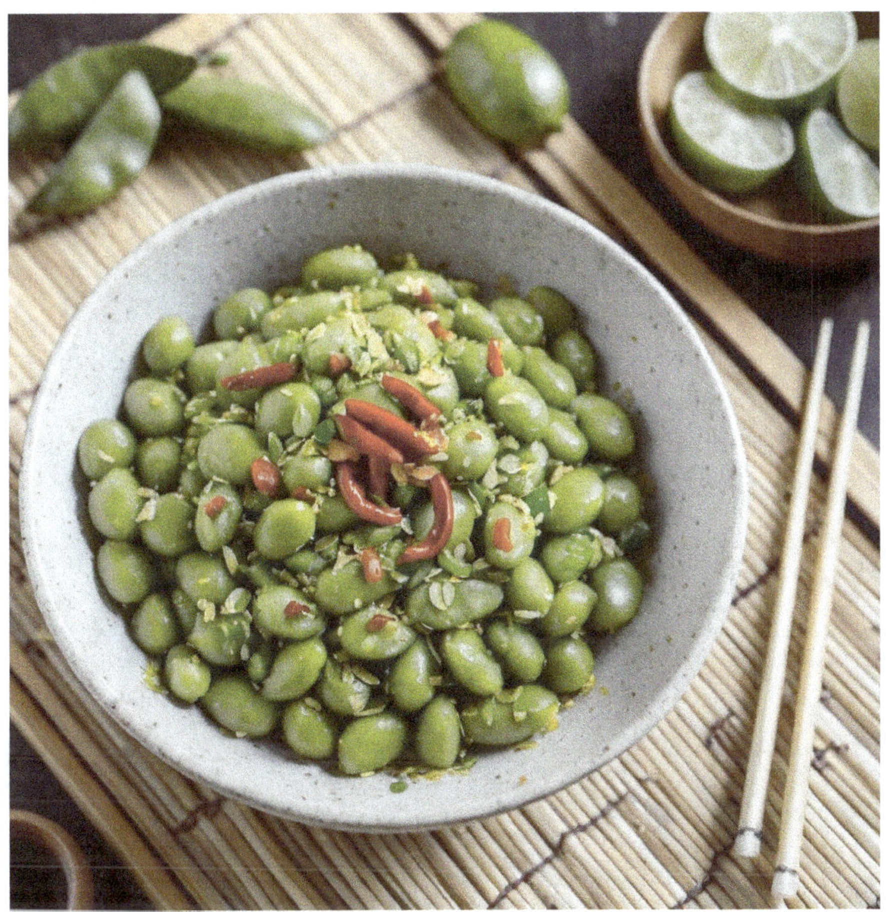

- **Yields:** 1 serving
- **Prep Time:** 5 minutes
- **Cook Time:** 5–7 minutes
- **Total Time:** 10–12 minutes

Ingredients:

- 1 cup fresh edamame pods (shelled or in pods)
- 1 teaspoon olive oil

- ½ teaspoon chili powder
- ½ tablespoon lime juice
- Pinch of salt

Instructions:

1. Bring a pot of salted water to a boil.
2. If using edamame pods, rinse and blanch them in boiling water for 2-3 minutes. Alternatively, steam fresh shelled edamame for 5-7 minutes.
3. Drain the edamame and transfer them to a bowl.
4. Drizzle with olive oil, chili powder, lime juice, and salt. Toss to coat.
5. Serve immediately while warm.

Tips:

- You can adjust the amount of chili powder to your spice preference.
- For a smoky flavor, use smoked paprika instead of chili powder.

* * *

Cucumber Yogurt Dip with Crudités

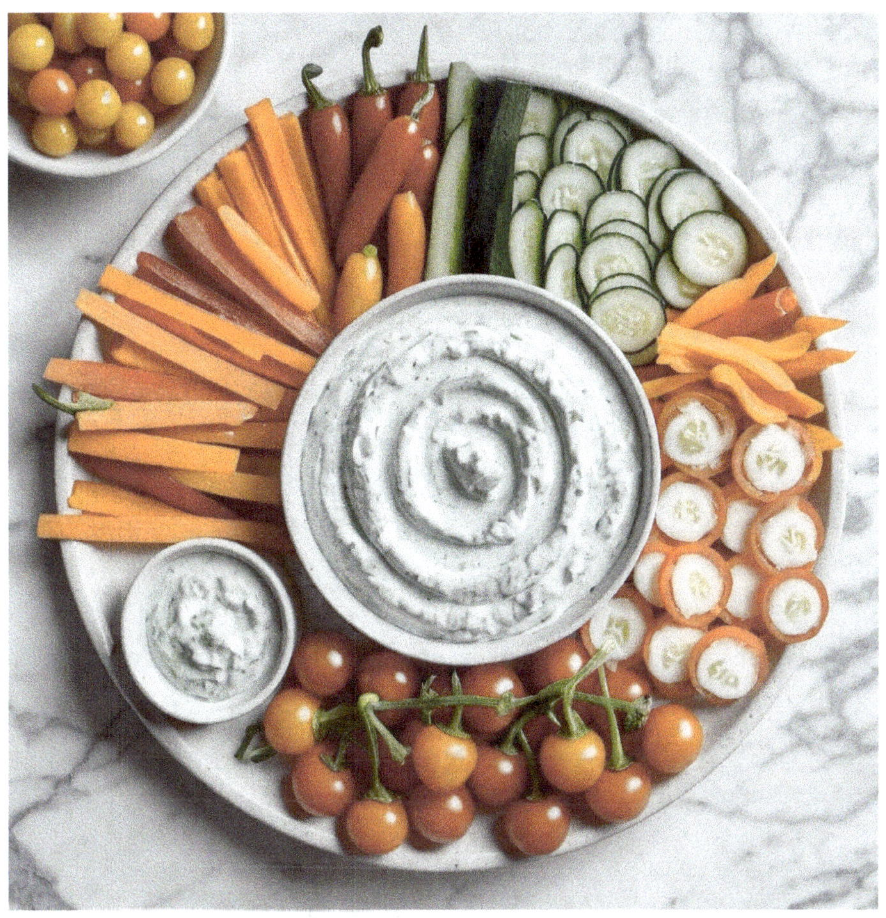

- **Yields:** 4 servings
- **Prep Time:** 10 minutes
- **Total Time:** 10 minutes

Ingredients:

- 1 cup lactose–free plain Greek yogurt
- ¼ cup chopped fresh dill
- 1 tablespoon lemon juice

- Pinch of salt
- 1 cucumber, sliced into sticks
- 1 red bell pepper, sliced into sticks
- Baby carrots (optional)

Instructions:

1. In a bowl, combine Greek yogurt, chopped dill, lemon juice, and salt. Stir well.
2. Wash and prepare the vegetables by slicing the cucumber and red bell pepper into sticks.
3. Serve the yogurt dip with the sliced cucumber, red bell pepper, and baby carrots (if using) for dipping.

Serving Suggestion:

For a more vibrant presentation, arrange the sliced vegetables on a platter with the yogurt dip in the center.

* * *

Rice Cake with Almond Butter and Sliced Banana

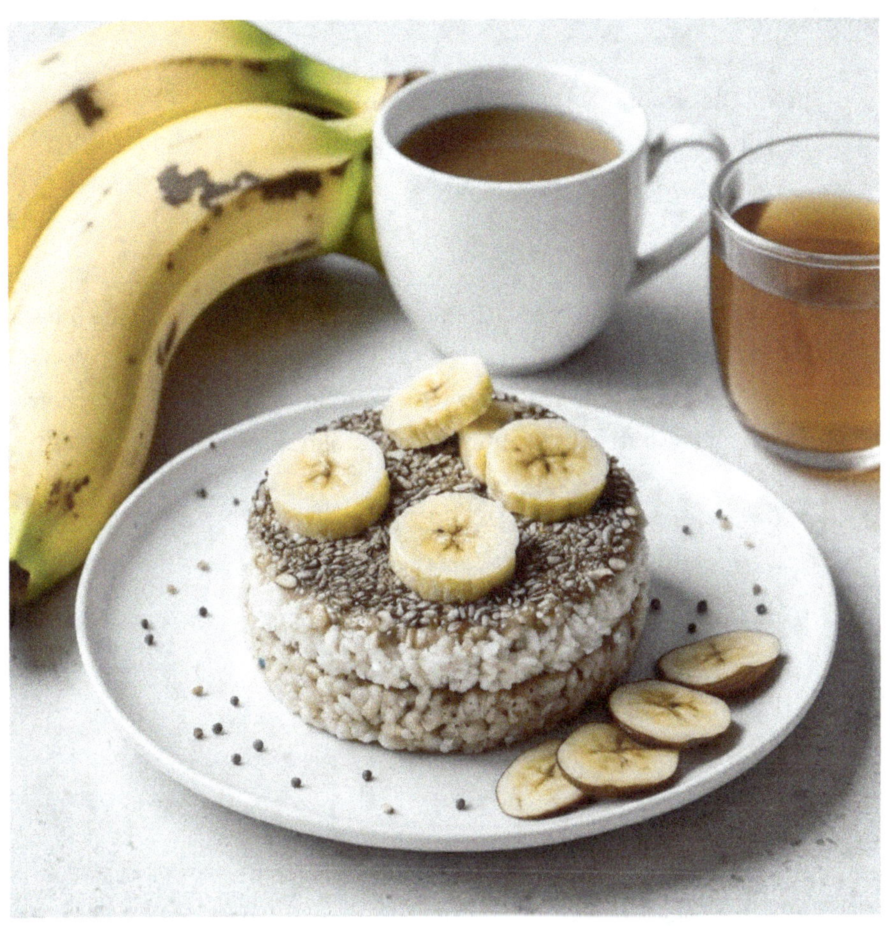

- **Yields:** 1 serving
- **Prep Time:** 2 minutes
- **Total Time:** 2 minutes

Ingredients:

- 1 rice cake
- 2 tablespoons almond butter
- ½ banana, sliced

Instructions:

1. Spread the almond butter evenly over the rice cake.
2. Top with sliced banana.

Tips:

- For a fun twist, use flavored rice cakes like cinnamon or chocolate (check FODMAP content).
- You can substitute almond butter with another nut butter of your choice, such as cashew butter or peanut butter (if tolerated).

* * *

Roasted Chickpeas with Herbs

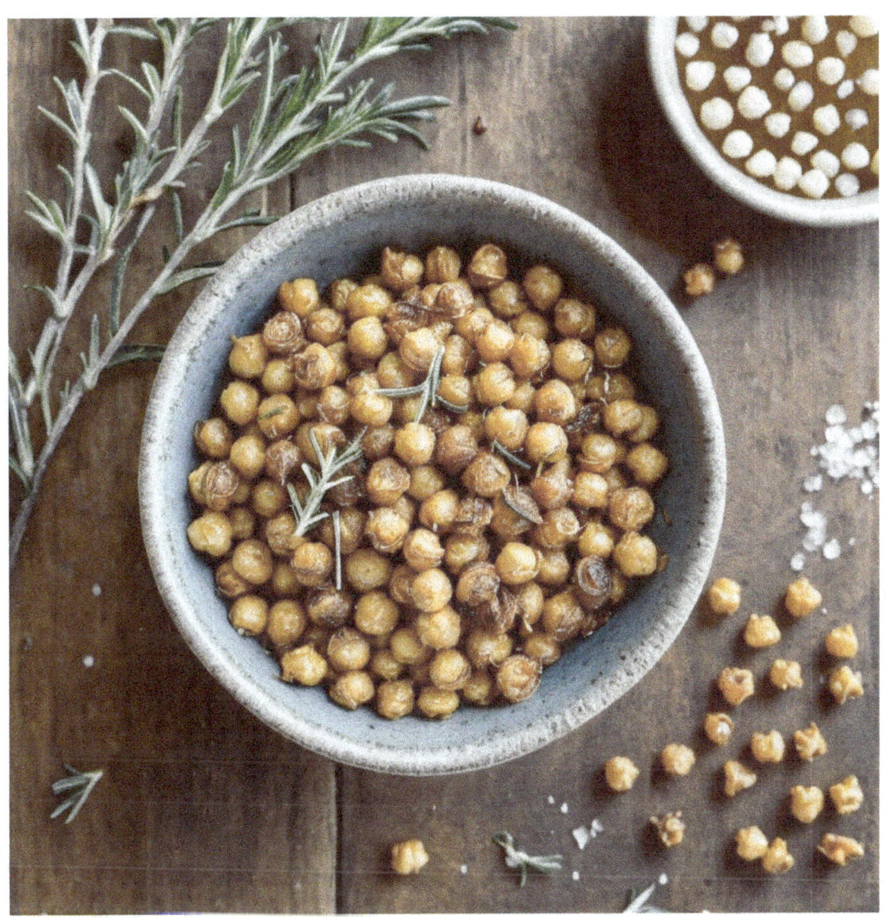

- **Yields:** 2-3 servings
- **Prep Time:** 5 minutes
- **Cook Time:** 20-25 minutes
- **Total Time:** 25-30 minutes

Ingredients:

- 1 (15 oz) can chickpeas, rinsed and drained
- 1 tablespoon olive oil

- ½ teaspoon dried oregano
- ½ teaspoon paprika
- Pinch of salt

Instructions:

1. Preheat oven to 400°F (200°C). Line a baking sheet with parchment paper.
2. Pat the drained chickpeas dry with a paper towel to ensure they crisp up properly.
3. In a bowl, toss the chickpeas with olive oil, oregano, paprika, and salt.
4. Spread the seasoned chickpeas on the prepared baking sheet in a single layer.
5. Roast for 20-25 minutes, or until golden brown and crispy, stirring occasionally.
6. Let cool slightly before serving.

Serving Suggestion:

Enjoy the roasted chickpeas as a standalone snack or sprinkle them over salads for added protein and crunch.

* * *

Baked Apples with Cinnamon and Walnuts

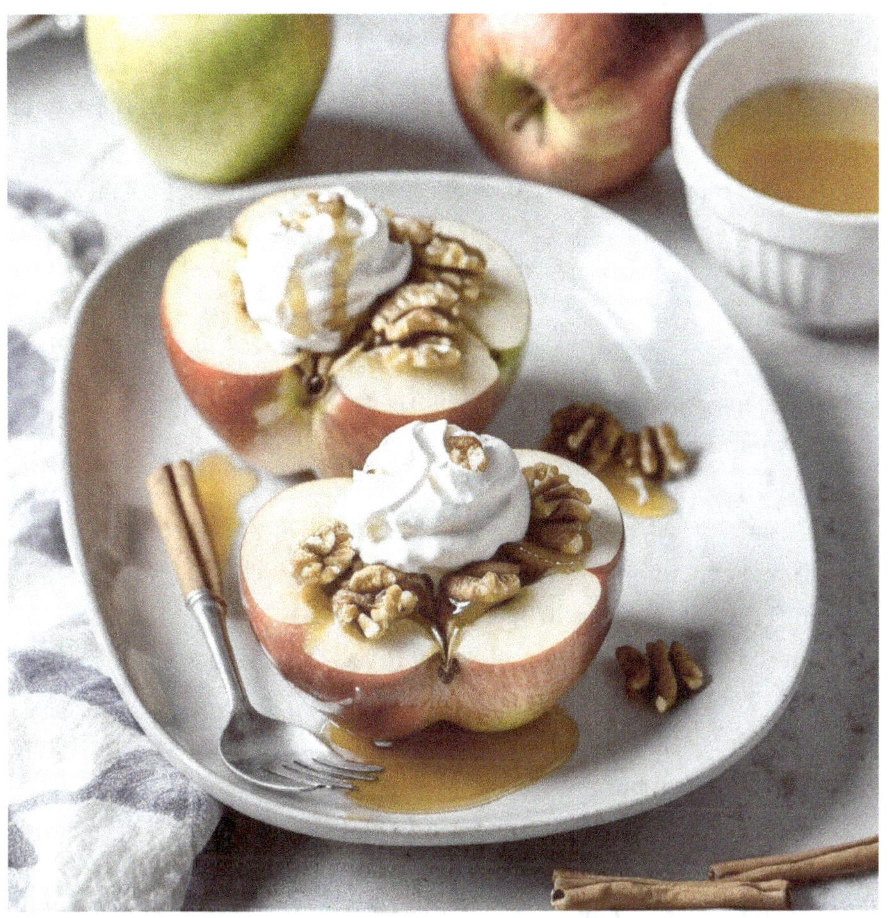

- **Yields:** 2 servings
- **Prep Time:** 10 minutes
- **Cook Time:** 30-35 minutes
- **Total Time:** 40-45 minutes

Ingredients:

- 2 apples (tart varieties like Granny Smith or Gala work well)
- ¼ cup chopped walnuts

- 1 tablespoon brown sugar (optional)
- 1 teaspoon ground cinnamon
- ½ tablespoon lactose-free butter, softened (or substitute with coconut oil)
- Optional toppings: Lactose-free whipped cream, vanilla ice cream (check FODMAP content)

Instructions:

1. Preheat oven to 375°F (190°C). Lightly grease a baking dish.
2. Wash and core the apples, leaving about ½ inch of flesh around the bottom.
3. In a small bowl, combine chopped walnuts, brown sugar (if using), and ground cinnamon.
4. Stuff the apple cores with the walnut mixture.
5. Dot the top of each apple with a pat of lactose-free butter (or coconut oil).
6. Pour a small amount of water (about ¼ cup) into the bottom of the baking dish to prevent burning.
7. Bake for 30–35 minutes, or until the apples are tender when pierced with a fork.
8. Let cool slightly before serving.

Serving Suggestion:

Top the baked apples with a dollop of lactose-free whipped cream or a scoop of vanilla ice cream (check FODMAP content) for an extra treat.

* * *

Dark Chocolate and Almond Bark

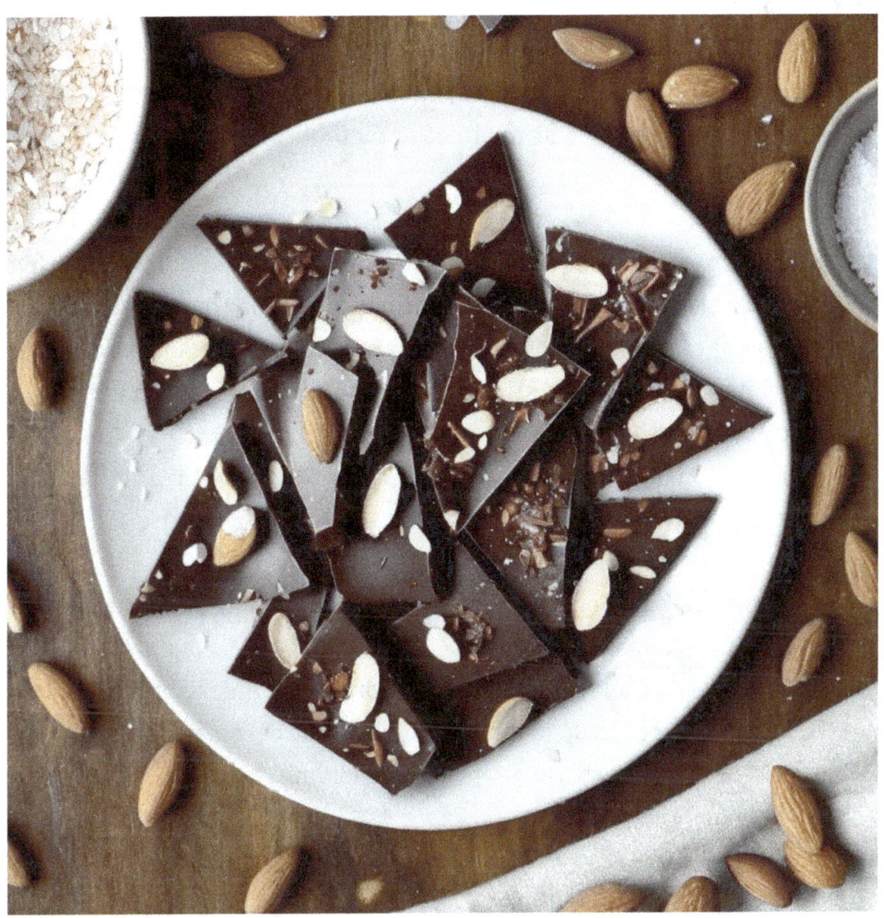

- **Yields:** 4-6 servings
- **Prep Time:** 10 minutes
- **Total Time:** 30 minutes (including chilling)

Ingredients:

- 6 ounces dark chocolate (at least 70% cacao), chopped
- ½ cup chopped almonds

Instructions:

1. Line a baking sheet with parchment paper.
2. Using a double boiler or microwave method, melt the chopped dark chocolate.

- **Double Boiler Method:** Fill a saucepan with a few inches of water. Bring the water to a simmer. Place a heat-resistant bowl on top of the saucepan, ensuring the bottom of the bowl doesn't touch the water. Add the chopped chocolate to the bowl and stir constantly until melted and smooth.
- **Microwave Method:** Place the chopped chocolate in a microwave-safe bowl. Heat on medium power for 30-second intervals, stirring after each interval, until melted and smooth.

1. Pour the melted chocolate onto the prepared baking sheet and spread evenly using a spatula.
2. Immediately sprinkle the chopped almonds over the melted chocolate.
3. Refrigerate for at least 30 minutes, or until the chocolate is set.
4. Break the chocolate bark into pieces for serving.

Tips:

- You can substitute chopped peanuts or other low-FODMAP nuts for the almonds (check FODMAP content).
- For a fun twist, drizzle melted white chocolate over the dark chocolate after spreading it on the baking sheet.

* * *

Coconut Chia Seed Pudding

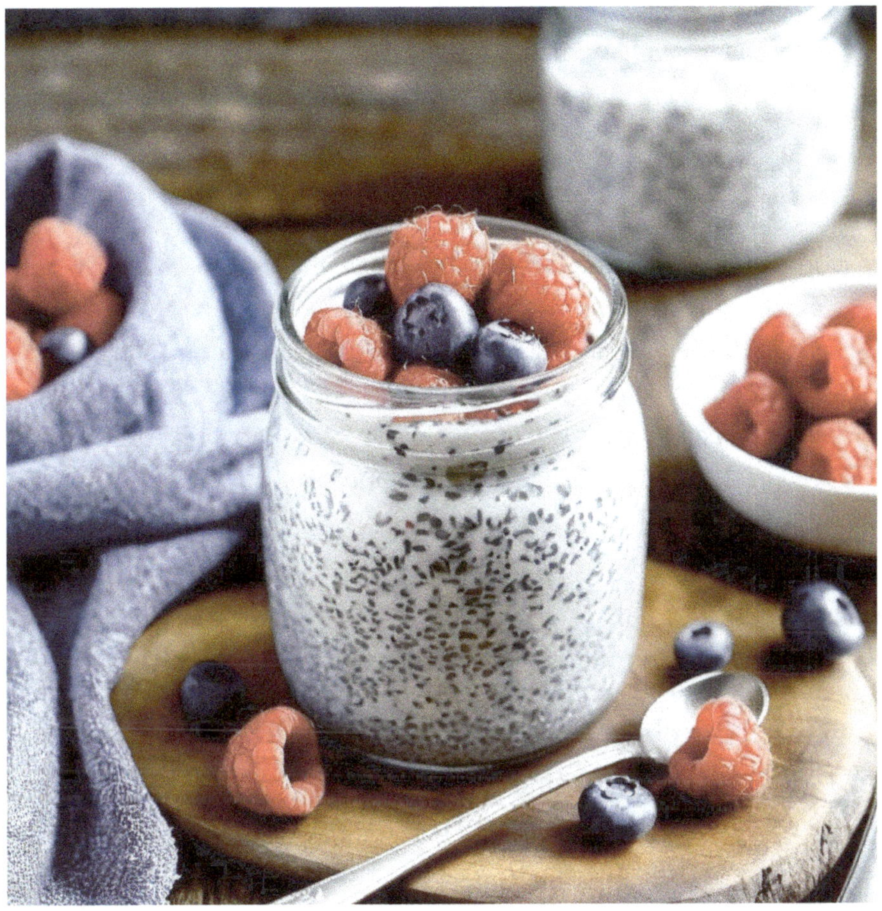

- **Yields:** 2–3 servings
- **Prep Time:** 5 minutes
- **Chill Time:** At least 2 hours, or overnight
- **Total Time:** 2+ hours

Ingredients:

- 1 cup canned coconut milk (full-fat)
- ½ cup chia seeds
- ½ teaspoon vanilla extract
- Optional toppings: Fresh berries, chopped nuts, shredded coconut

Instructions:

1. In a bowl or jar, whisk together the coconut milk, chia seeds, and vanilla extract.
2. Cover the bowl or jar and refrigerate for at least 2 hours, or overnight, for the chia seeds to absorb the liquid and thicken the pudding.
3. When ready to serve, stir the pudding well. Top with fresh berries, chopped nuts, or shredded coconut (optional).

Tips:

- For a thicker pudding, use a 3:1 ratio of chia seeds to coconut milk (¾ cup chia seeds and ½ cup coconut milk).
- You can experiment with different flavors by adding a pinch of ground cinnamon, nutmeg, or a few drops of stevia to the pudding mixture.

* * *

Low-FODMAP Fruit Smoothie

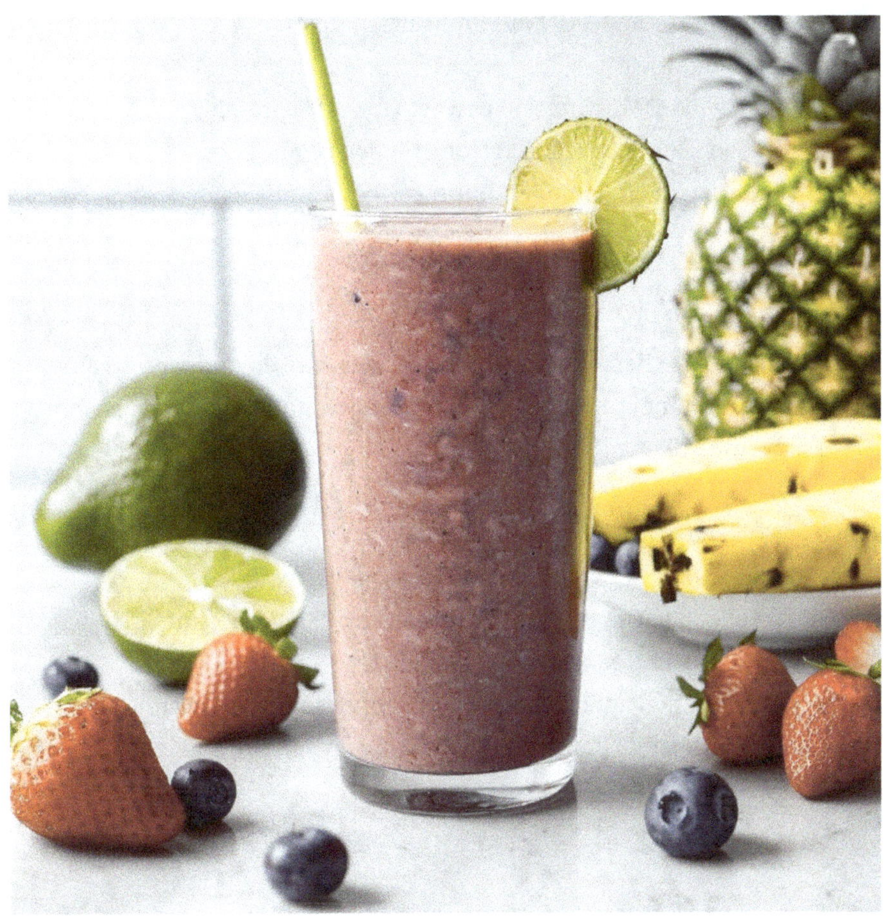

- **Yields:** 1 serving
- **Prep Time:** 5 minutes
- **Total Time:** 5 minutes

Ingredients:

- ½ cup frozen low–FODMAP berries (blueberries, raspberries)
- ¼ cup chopped banana (unripe for lower FODMAP content)
- ½ cup lactose-free yogurt (or coconut milk)

- ½ cup water (or low-FODMAP milk alternative)
- Optional additions:
- 1 scoop low-FODMAP protein powder (for extra protein)
- 1 tablespoon chopped spinach (for a hidden veggie boost)
- Pinch of ground cinnamon or nutmeg (for extra flavor)

Instructions:

1. Blend all ingredients together in a blender until smooth and creamy.
2. Add more water or milk alternative if desired for a thinner consistency.
3. Enjoy immediately!

Tips:

- Feel free to experiment with different low-FODMAP fruits like mango, pineapple (in limited quantities), or kiwi.
- Frozen fruits add a thicker and colder consistency to the smoothie. You can use fresh fruits if preferred, but you may need to add ice cubes for a chilled drink.

* * *

Baked Pears with Ginger and Honey

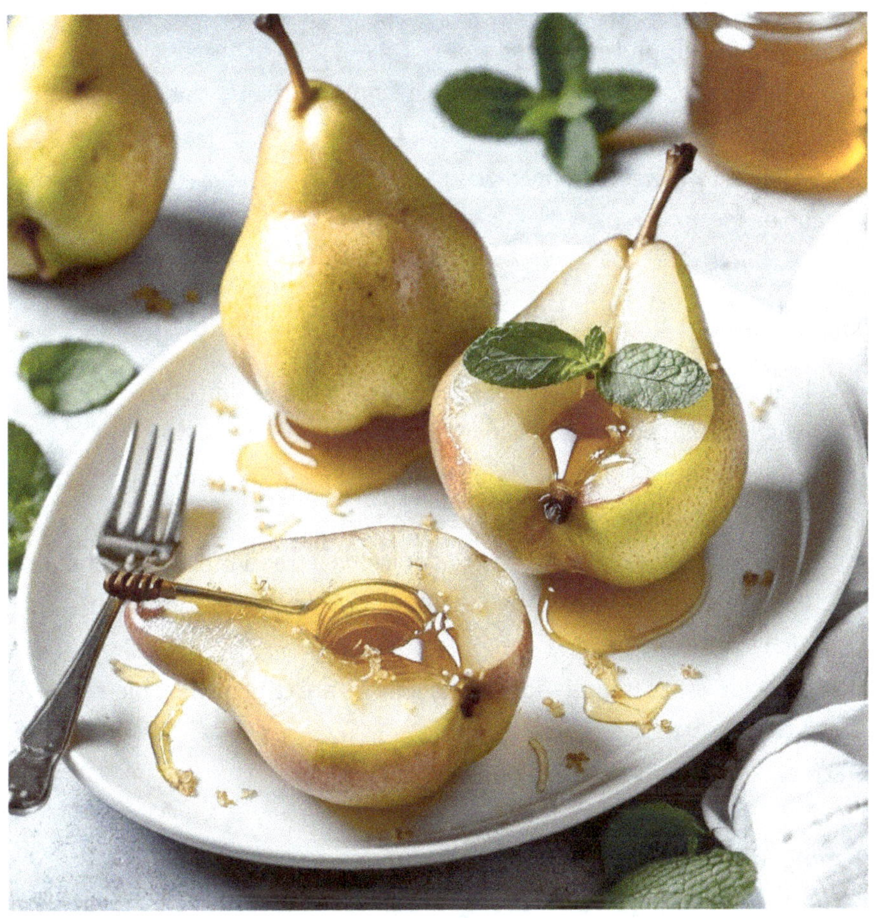

- **Yields:** 2 servings
- **Prep Time:** 10 minutes
- **Cook Time:** 30-35 minutes
- **Total Time:** 40-45 minutes

Ingredients:

- 2 ripe pears (Bosc or Bartlett varieties work well)
- 1 tablespoon chopped fresh ginger

- 1 tablespoon honey
- 1 teaspoon ground cinnamon
- ½ tablespoon lactose-free butter, softened (or substitute with coconut oil)
- Optional toppings: Chopped walnuts, crumbled lactose-free gingersnap cookies

Instructions:

1. Preheat oven to 375°F (190°C). Lightly grease a baking dish.
2. Wash and core the pears, leaving the stem intact.
3. In a small bowl, combine chopped ginger, honey, and ground cinnamon.
4. Stuff the pear cores with the ginger mixture.
5. Dot the top of each pear with a pat of lactose-free butter (or coconut oil).
6. Pour a small amount of water (about ¼ cup) into the bottom of the baking dish to prevent burning.
7. Bake for 30-35 minutes, or until the pears are tender when pierced with a fork.
8. Let cool slightly before serving.

Serving Suggestion:

Top the baked pears with chopped walnuts and crumbled lactose-free gingersnap cookies for added texture and flavor.

Maintaining a Low-FODMAP Lifestyle

Living with IBS and following a low-FODMAP diet can be a transformative journey. While the initial reintroduction phase can be challenging, the long-term benefits of managing your IBS symptoms are worth the effort. This chapter will equip you with strategies for maintaining a successful low-FODMAP lifestyle, addressing potential challenges, and prioritizing your overall gut health.

Long-Term Success with Low-FODMAP:

- **Gradual Reintroduction:** After completing the elimination phase, it's crucial to follow a structured reintroduction plan under the guidance of a healthcare professional. This allows you to identify your individual FODMAP triggers and gradually reintroduce tolerated FODMAPs back into your diet.

- **Planning and Preparation:** Meal planning and prepping low-FODMAP staples can become a valuable habit for long-term success. Utilize low-FODMAP cookbooks, online resources, and grocery shopping lists to stay on track.

- **Embrace Low-FODMAP Cooking:** Learning to cook low-FODMAP meals at home empowers you to manage your diet while still enjoying delicious and satisfying food. Experiment with new recipes and discover the variety of low-FODMAP options available.

- **Mindful Eating:** Pay attention to your body's hunger and fullness cues. Eat slowly and savor your food to promote better digestion and avoid overeating.

- **Maintain a Food Journal:** Keeping a food journal can help you track potential triggers, IBS symptoms, and overall well-being. This information can be valuable for discussions with your healthcare professional.

Dealing with Challenges and Setbacks:

- **Social Situations:** Navigate social gatherings and dining out by planning ahead. Bring low-FODMAP snacks if necessary, and communicate your dietary needs politely to friends, family, and restaurant staff.
- **Travel:** Pack low-FODMAP staples and research restaurants or grocery stores at your destination beforehand. Consider bringing a cooler bag for transporting food if needed.
- **Emotional Eating:** Identify and address emotional triggers that might lead to unhealthy eating habits. Relaxation techniques such as deep breathing or meditation can be helpful tools.
- **Setbacks Happen:** Don't be discouraged by occasional slip-ups. The key is to learn from them, get back on track, and maintain a positive attitude.

The Importance of Gut Health and Stress Management:

- **The Gut Microbiome:** A healthy gut microbiome plays a vital role in digestion, nutrient absorption, and overall well-being. Following a low-FODMAP diet can help create a favorable environment for beneficial gut bacteria to flourish.
- **Stress Management:** Chronic stress can exacerbate IBS symptoms. Prioritize stress-management techniques like yoga, meditation, or spending time in nature to promote gut health and overall well-being.
- **Adequate Sleep:** Aim for 7-8 hours of quality sleep each night. Adequate sleep allows your body to rest and repair, which can positively impact your gut health and IBS management.
- **Regular Exercise:** Regular physical activity can improve gut motility, reduce stress, and promote overall health. Choose exercises you enjoy and incorporate them into your routine.

Remember, maintaining a low-FODMAP lifestyle is a journey, not a destination. By incorporating these strategies and prioritizing your gut health, you can empower yourself to manage your IBS and live a fulfilling life.

Conclusion

Congratulations! You've embarked on a journey of managing your IBS and reclaiming control of your well-being through the low-FODMAP diet. This cookbook has equipped you with delicious recipes, essential information, and practical strategies to navigate your low-FODMAP lifestyle with confidence.

Remember, a healthy diet is just one piece of the puzzle. Prioritize stress management, adequate sleep, and regular exercise for a holistic approach to gut health. As you continue your low-FODMAP journey, embrace the opportunity to discover new low-FODMAP favorites and rediscover the joy of cooking and eating. Let this be the beginning of a flavorful future filled with delicious, nourishing meals!